W0037469

TRANSACTIONS

of the

AMERICAN PHILOSOPHICAL SOCIETY

Volume 89, Pt. 1

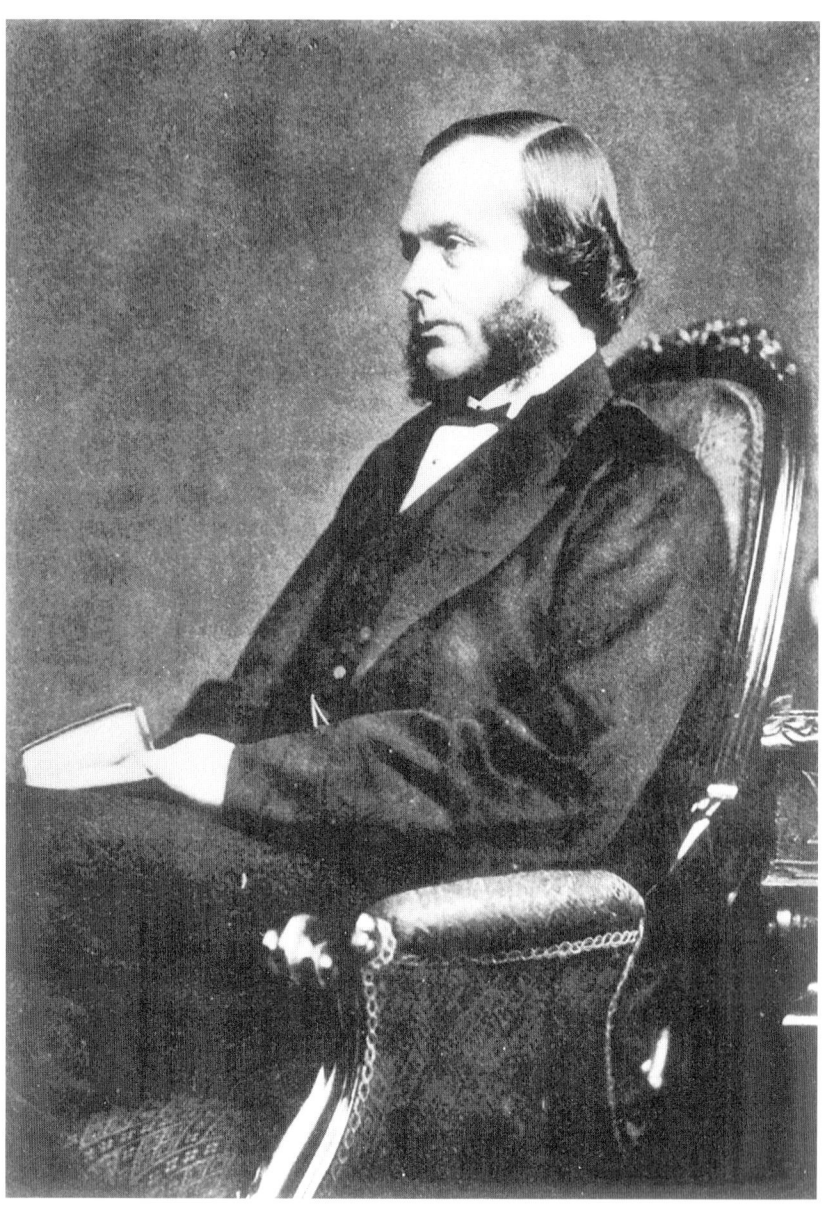

Joseph Lister

TRANSACTIONS

of the

AMERICAN PHILOSOPHICAL SOCIETY

Held at Philadelphia

For Promoting Useful Knowledge

Volume 89, Pt. 1

"A Time to Heal": The Diffusion of Listerism in Victorian Britain

JERRY L. GAW

Associate Professor of History
Lipscomb University

American Philosophical Society
Independence Square • Philadelphia
1999

Copyright © 1999 by the American Philosophical Society for its *Transactions* series, Volume 89. All rights reserved.

Library of Congress Cataloging-in-Publication Data

Gaw, Jerry L., 1952–
    A time to heal : the diffusion of Listerism in Victorian Britain / Jerry L. Gaw.
      p.   cm. — (Transactions of the American Philosophical Society ; v. 89,
  pt. 1 <1999–   >)
    Includes bibliographical references and index.
    ISBN 0-87169-891-9 (pbk.)
    1. Medicine—Great Britain—History—19th century.   2. Surgery—
Great Britain—History—19th century.   3. Medical innovations—Great
Britain—History—19th century.   4. Surgery, Aseptic and antiseptic—
History.   5. Diffusion of innovations—Great Britain—History—19th
century.   I. Title.   II. Series.
R487.G39   1999
610′.941′09034—dc21   99-19605
                                                                        CIP

ISBN:0-87169-891-9
US ISSN:0065-9746

For Ralph,
an example as a Christian and as a man

CONTENTS

List of Illustrations[*]

[*] All illustrations come from the National Library of Medicine in Bethesda, Maryland, except Figures 8 and 13, which are reproduced by kind permission of the President and Council of the Royal College of Surgeons of England.

Acknowledgments

An undertaking such as this would be impossible without the assistance of many selfless individuals who willingly contribute their wisdom, talents, time, and unwavering support. The idea was conceived in the fertile mind of C. James Haug, Professor of History at Mississippi State University. He also tightened the prose and clarified many of the arguments. The successful completion of the work is largely due to his encouragement and optimism. Research for the book was facilitated by Mary Teloh, Special Collections Librarian for the History of Medicine at the Eskind Biomedical Library of Vanderbilt University. Her pleasant and cooperative manner made an arduous task much more tolerable. She granted access to nineteenth-century medical journals and other primary sources, and her permission to photocopy those that were not too fragile is remembered with particular appreciation.

Others who rendered invaluable aid were Alison Stevenson, Assistant Librarian and Archivist at the Royal College of Surgeons of Edinburgh; Claire Jackson, Archivist at the Royal College of Surgeons of England; and Richard Aspin, Curator of the Western Manuscripts Collection at the Wellcome Institute for the History of Medicine. They not only provided what was requested but also suggested additional materials which were very helpful. The staff of Lipscomb University's Beaman Library also assisted in the research, especially in locating sources through interlibrary loan; Marie Byers, Jonna Devar, Carolyn Wilson, Judy Butler, and Deneen Ferrell willingly and promptly found what was needed. Kim Reed, Assistant Professor of Foreign Languages at Lipscomb, graciously agreed to translate three letters from Louis Pasteur to Joseph Lister and did so as a professional courtesy for a colleague. Another fellow faculty member, Kent Clinger, Associate Professor of Chemistry, shared his expertise by describing certain compounds and verifying the accuracy of several definitions in the Glossary.

Two Vice-Presidents of Academic Affairs and the Provost at Lipscomb allocated funds for photocopying, purchasing hard to find sources, and overseas travel. Earl Dennis, James T. Arnett, and W. Craig Bledsoe were more than generous with the Faculty Research and Development Grants at their disposal. The members of the Department of History and Political Science at Lipscomb, past and present, offered unceasing moral support, even when the department's printer was commandeered. Robert E. Hooper and James Lee McDonough set the example by continuing to research, write, and publish while performing their many other academic responsibilities. Tim Johnson and Richard Goode commiserated as they worked on manuscripts of their own for publication. Dwight Tays, David Lawrence, Don Cole, Guy Vanderpool, and Neal Allison expressed genuine interest in the project during various stages of its development. The secretaries, Joann Harwell and Jennie Johnson, did not hesitate to make copies and prepare drafts for mailing, often on short notice.

Special thanks goes to Walton Beacham for allowing portions of a chapter on Joseph Lister, from volume seven of his *Research Guide to European Historical Biography,* to be reproduced. Almost all of the Chronology and the Review Essay came from that entry. Gratitude is also extended to Carole Lefaivre-Rochester of the American Philosophical Society for her skill and knowledge as an editor. She thoroughly explained the changes that had to be made, implemented them judiciously, and was always approachable. Furthermore, Richard M. Krause, M.D., Senior Scientific Advisor at the Fogarty International Center of the National Institutes of Health, was kind enough to read the study and offered many constructive comments for improving it.

Finally, the sacrifices a family makes to insure the fruition of such a venture are legion, and it is with deepest love for Vicki, my wife, and David, my son, that these acknowledgments end. Her faith never flagged, and the desire to finish for his sake kept motivation high. It was not for prestige that this endeavor was begun, but in order to have a better life. Though the effort is over, the satisfaction of achieving it remains. Obviously, a number of people were involved in the realization of this goal, but any errors are the sole responsibility of the author.

INTRODUCTION

THE WISE MAN, SOLOMON, once said that there is "a time to every purpose under the heaven," and his list included "a time to heal."[1] Nineteenth-century Britain was rife with new concepts that furthered the political, military, social, economic, intellectual, and religious aims of individuals and governments. Nationalism, imperialism, Romanticism, liberalism, Darwinism, and higher criticism are just a few in a century defined by them. Less well known is Listerism, but it had a greater impact on Victorian society than all of the above. It touched the daily lives of people in a positive way by mending their bodies and giving them hope, and it engendered faith in an establishment that had become increasingly ineffective in winning their trust.

That establishment was the medical community, and it naturally lends itself to an analysis of the synthesis that results from the challenge to its traditions by innovation. Along with religious and military organizations, it is historically one of the institutions of society most resistant to change. Diffusion studies in the area of medical sociology have either focused on innovative techniques that practitioners have assimilated or inventive ideas that the public has accepted. The latter has usually taken place when the medical establishment has espoused new doctrines as aggressively as previously held dogmas in order to influence popular opinion. The former has typically happened without subsequent campaigns to sway public thinking and with little or no impact on the conservatism of the profession.[2]

Certain factors affecting whether or not the medical profession has incorporated imaginative methods have been documented, and they help elucidate why there has been so much reluctance to embrace new knowledge. A 1966 inquiry into the adoption of an experimental drug by physicians revealed a host of considerations that determined their decisions. Educational background, type of practice, contact with members of the profession from other locales, attendance at conferences, patients' attitudes, the impact of opinions expressed in medical journals, and the amount of information to be digested about a particular novelty were all cited as discernible criteria.[3]

The facts relating to the 1966 study were just as important a century earlier when the diffusion of antisepsis began. Surgeons in county and provincial areas responded more positively to Joseph Lister's technique than those in cities because infectious diseases were much easier to control in small hospitals and private homes. This was especially true of ovariotomists, even in urban settings, because many of them worked out of their own houses and did not encounter the problem of cross-infection which was common in metropolitan hospitals.[4] Where surgeons had studied medicine was

---

[1] Ecclesiastes 3:1–8 KJV

[2] Everett M. Rogers, *Diffusion of Innovations* (New York: The Free Press, 1962), p. 45.

[3] James S. Coleman, Elihu Katz, and Herbert Menzel, *Medical Innovation: A Diffusion Study* (Indianapolis: The Bobbs-Merrill Company, Inc., 1966), pp. 7–17, 40–44, 157–79.

[4] Elaine Larson, "Innovations in Health Care: Antisepsis as a Case Study," *American Journal of Public Health* 79 (January 1989): 95–96; John Shepherd, "Lister and the Development of Abdominal Surgery," in *Medicine and Science in the 1860s,* ed. F. N. L. Poynter (London: Wellcome Institute of [now known and hereafter cited as "for"] the History of Medicine, 1968), p. 109.

1

another element in their willingness to consider the antiseptic method. Those who were educated on the Continent or in Scotland received scientific instruction, while those schooled in England were taught a philosophical approach to healing. Peer pressure, exerted at annual meetings and in the medical press, also must have kept some from trying Lister's system. Finally, there was a great deal of information about his system to understand, and most surgeons at large hospitals simply did not take the time to thoroughly investigate it.[5]

Each of these components played a role in the diffusion of Listerism, but it was adopted because its success was greater and more consistent than other methods of healing the sick. The circumstances which made this possible were a theory for explaining the consistency, scientific evidence to support the theory, and a courageous person who was capable of bringing about the necessary changes, even if it meant risking personal and professional alienation. That person was Joseph Lister.

---

[5] Joseph Ben-David, "Roles and Innovations in Medicine," *The American Journal of Sociology* 65 (May 1960): 557–64.

1. Medical Administration as a Factor in the Diffusion of Listerism

In 1854 the British entered the Crimean War, which claimed many more lives from surgical diseases than weapons; that same year Joseph Lister began his medical career, assisting in the wards of the Edinburgh Royal Infirmary. The medical profession experienced "a sort of fatalism" because of its inability to significantly reduce mortality rates following surgery, but it became such a source of "grief and mental worry" to Lister that he developed "a sense of discontent with things as they were."[1] He had gone to Scotland on the advice of William Sharpey, his physiology professor at University College in London. Sharpey knew James Syme, a famous teacher of clinical surgery at the University of Edinburgh who was generally viewed as the greatest surgeon in the United Kingdom. Sharpey himself was one of many English surgeons who had sought training in Scotland after John Hunter had elevated the status of surgery as an occupation.[2]

Hunter had taught Edward Jenner and is looked upon as the first surgeon to take a scientific approach to the study of medicine. Unlike other surgeons, he based his medical practice on physiology and pathology, providing him with insights into healing the human body that had eluded more specialized researchers. His 1794 *A Treatise on the Blood, Inflammation, and Gunshot Wounds*, for example, was the first systematic study of swelling that had ever been done. In it he showed how inflammation was common to all diseases. He also experimented with the transplantation of tissues, performed the first successful artificial insemination in a human, and provided the initial demonstration of the principle of collateral circulation.

Largely due to Hunter's work, surgery became a respected profession, not the hobby of barbers. Since the universities in Scotland taught medicine and surgery from Hunter's scientific perspective, students who wanted to emulate him journeyed north.[3] Lister patterned himself after Hunter more than most did; some of his earliest researches after he began his medical practice dealt with the causes of inflammation and coagulation. He determined that the two conditions stemmed from the same type of chemical changes, the only difference being that the former occurred in the tissues while the later obviously took place in the blood.[4] Fifty years after he started studying inflammation, Lister twice credited the inquiry with being "an indispensable preliminary to that on antiseptic surgery."[5]

Scottish universities had several other characteristics that distinguished them from

---

[1] James G. Mumford, *Surgical Memoirs and Other Essays* (New York: Moffat, Yard & Company, 1908), pp. 101–104.
[2] A. J. Youngson, *The Scientific Revolution in Victorian Medicine* (New York: Holmes & Meier Publishers, Inc., 1979), p. 138.
[3] Howard W. Haggard, *The Doctor in History* (New York: Dorset Press, 1989), pp. 320–21; Sherwin B. Nuland, *Doctors: The Biography of Medicine* (New York: Alfred A. Knopf, 1988), pp. 185–86, 188–89.
[4] Richard B. Fisher, *Joseph Lister, 1827–1912* (New York: Stein and Day, 1977), pp. 70–72, 83–93.
[5] Joseph Lister to Hector Clare Cameron, 19 February 1907, Joseph Lister Papers, Library, Royal College of Surgeons of Edinburgh, Edinburgh, GD5, 67.

their sister institutions to the south. Their schools of medicine were founded on scholarly tradition, whereas English medical education was dominated by hospitals and practitioners. Additionally, they did not require religious admission tests and were relatively inexpensive, which helps explain why they drew some of the best students in the United Kingdom. Even Oxford and Cambridge refused to stress the importance of original research, and their graduates did not have to pass an examination to obtain a medical license. Located in rural England, their laboratory facilities and clinical materials were also inadequate. Finally, the faculties of English universities tended to view surgery as a form of manual labor, not a respectable calling for academics.[6]

James Syme addressed the issue of licensing medical students in 1870, pointing out that graduates of the University of Edinburgh had to pass one examination in medicine and, after a minimum of three courses, another one in surgery. Clearly, the University of Edinburgh placed a great deal of emphasis on surgery, while English universities customarily ignored it. The clinical approach to medicine had been instituted at the University of Edinburgh by men trained in eighteenth-century Holland, the country considered to be the most medically advanced in the world at that time.[7]

Syme was familiar with English schools, having briefly taken a position at University College, London, in 1848. He and Sharpey became co-workers there. Syme began his duties in London the same year that Lister enrolled as a medical student at University College, but he stayed less than five months because of conflicts with the institution's Council which wanted him to oversee both the professorial chair in clinical surgery and the chair in systematic surgery. Syme was gone before Lister registered, in spite of the fact that he had been "cordially received by the heads of the medical profession as well as by the students, with whom he became very popular, and who 'invariably paid him great respect.'"[8]

Syme had been a clinical lecturer for two decades before he ever met Lister and had distinguished himself as a surgeon by attempting procedures that were much simpler than standard practices. He despised complicated surgical tools such as the chain saw, and refused to practice intricate procedures when less elaborate ones worked. He preferred to transfix skin flaps over an amputee's stump, so that they might adhere naturally, than to close the wound entirely and cover it with artificial adhesives. He also tried to excise diseased bones instead of amputating limbs. Prior to the advent of anesthesia, he made a name for himself as a surgeon by being the first in Scotland to perform an amputation at the hip-joint. Calling it "the greatest and bloodiest operation in surgery," he executed it in approximately one minute, speed being of the utmost importance. All the more amazing was the fact that he had never seen, much less assisted in, such an operation. Before he introduced this technique, legs were amputated in a more time-consuming, circular method at the top of the femur.[9] (See Figure 1.)

Amputations before anesthetics could best be described as butchery. Patients had to be restrained by as many as four assistants and were able to see the hideous instru-

[6] Gerald L. Geison, "Social and Institutional Factors in the Stagnancy of English Physiology, 1840–1870," *Bulletin of the History of Medicine* 46 (January-February 1972): 43–45, 56–57.
[7] James G. Wakley, "Mr. Syme on Medical Reform," *The Lancet* (15 January 1870): 89; Erwin Ackerknecht, *A Short History of Medicine,* rev. ed. (Baltimore: The Johns Hopkins University Press, 1982), p. 130.
[8] Alexander Miles, *The Edinburgh School of Surgery before Lister* (London: A. & C. Black, Ltd., 1918), pp. 193–94.
[9] Ibid., pp. 179–84, 189–90; Youngson, *Scientific Revolution,* p. 31.

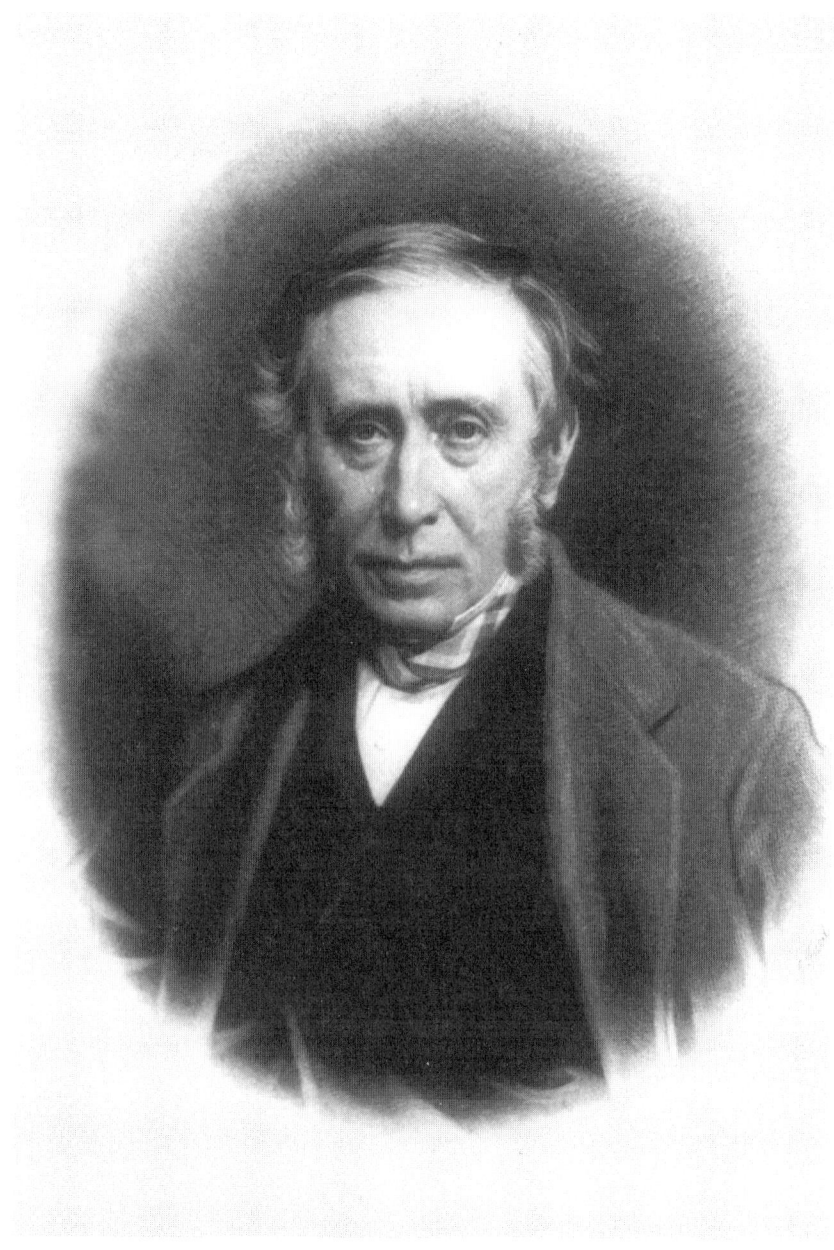

Figure 1. James Syme

ments that were being used. They screamed and frequently fainted from seeing their own blood spurt from their bodies, but the surgeon was not deterred from his task. On many occasions, an observer would time the surgeon in order to compare his speed with that of other cutters, and the fastest was much esteemed by all medical students. Robert Liston, who was Syme's cousin and taught him the flap transfixion method of healing stumps, was recognized as the quickest amputator in Great Britain; his record time for truncating a limb was twenty-five seconds. He also invented a longer, straighter knife, and arterial forceps for amputations.[10]

Liston had preceded Syme in the chair of surgery at the University of Edinburgh, from where he went to University College in London. Upon his unexpected death in 1847, only one year after performing the first surgery in England using anesthesia, he was again replaced by Syme. Lister was present when Liston administered ether in a London operating theater on December 21, 1846, and had probably attended some of his lectures. The application of ether to surgery had originally been publicly demonstrated at Boston's Massachusetts General Hospital two months earlier; the surgeon, John Warren, had been persuaded by a dentist, William Morton, to try anesthesia, and when it was successful Warren proclaimed that it was "no humbug." Liston is said to have introduced ether to Europe as "a Yankee dodge," but after he used it he exulted that it "beats mesmerism hollow."[11]

During an amputation Liston would hold the knife, which had just been used to lay open the skin, with his teeth in order to keep his hands free for surgery. His most spectacular case, though, resulted in the deaths of three individuals. Following one amputation, which lasted less than two and a half minutes, the patient died from gangrene. While operating, Liston had accidentally severed the fingers of one of his assistants, who also died from gangrene. A third individual, who was merely observing, expired from hysteria, thinking that Liston had punctured his internal organs when only his coat had been cut.[12]

Syme's notoriety was not based primarily on speed, although his hip-joint technique was extremely fast. His renown centered around the development of an amputation at the ankle-joint that still bears his name and is looked upon as the most effective surgical procedure in its specialty to this day. It replaced amputations below the knee, which had been routine for incurable ankle diseases, and provided the patient with an appendage capable of supporting the body's weight. Syme's innovation was the crowning accomplishment that assured his place in medical history regardless of his other contributions.

Certainly, Lister's willingness to examine new possibilities can be attributed in large part to Syme's influence on him, though Syme was not always receptive to new techniques. If they originated through the work of non-surgeons, he was particularly

[10] H. Laing Gordon, *Sir James Young Simpson and Chloroform (1811–1870)* (London: T. Fisher Unwin, 1897), pp. 89–90; Miles, *Edinburgh School*, pp. 161, 165–66.

[11] Miles, *Edinburgh School*, pp. 162–64, 167; Fisher, *Joseph Lister*, pp. 36–37, 40; W. J. Bishop, *The Early History of Surgery* (New York: Barnes & Noble, Inc., 1960), pp. 160–61, 166; mesmerism is named for Anton Mesmer (d. 1815), who conceived of what became the most recognized method of anesthetizing people psychologically in European history. Lois Magner, *A History of Medicine* (New York: Marcel Dekker, Inc., 1992), p. 282.

[12] Richard Gordon, *Great Medical Disasters* (New York: Stein and Day, 1983; reprint ed., New York: Dorset Press, 1986), pp. 19–21.

obstinate. For example, he was unjustifiably hesitant to use anesthetics because James Y. Simpson, the discoverer of chloroform, was a professor of midwifery at the University of Edinburgh. As one writer noted, "His adoption of anesthesia was delayed more because the discovery emanated from the obstetrical department than because he failed to appreciate its advantages."[13]

Lister, like Syme, chose to enter medicine as a surgeon, but in the mid-nineteenth century the distinctions that separated physicians, surgeons, and apothecaries were far from clear. Members of the three professions battled one another over issues related to professional status and responsibilities. Before 1858 the British medical profession was approaching a state of utter confusion. Licenses to practice medicine were granted by nineteen different agencies, and they did not all follow the same regulations. Some practitioners held degrees and licenses, while others had neither. There was no way to control quackery or the peddling of drugs. Three organizations loosely oversaw the separate medical fields. These were the Royal College of Physicians, the Royal College of Surgeons, and the Society of Apothecaries.

Although the first of these organizations predated the others by three centuries, physicians composed only five percent of the total number of English practitioners in 1850. In 1847, for example, England had six hundred and eighty-three physicians, three-fourths of whom lived in London. The Royal College of Surgeons, on the other hand, boasted approximately eight thousand members by the middle of the nineteenth century, but physicians viewed surgeons as craftsmen who had entered a guild through apprenticeship rather than as philosophers who had studied medicine at institutions of higher learning. Physicians also considered apothecaries to be tradesmen, even though the Apothecaries Act of 1815 allowed them to practice surgery as well as general medicine. Moreover, the act required all medical men who prescribed or dispensed drugs to take the License of the Society of Apothecaries regardless of what other license they might hold. Like surgeons, apothecaries became qualified through apprenticeship, and in 1834 six thousand certified pharmacists practiced their profession in England.[14]

Enormous differences in status existed among the three professions. As Frederick F. Cartwright wrote in his masterful *The Development of Modern Surgery,* the function of an apothecary was

> as a kind of general practitioner who dispensed his own medicines. The proud physician, a man of education and learned in the classics, was primarily interested in diagnosis. He therefore tended to deal with the type of disease which cannot be detected by superficial examination; overt disease he regarded as the province of the surgeon.[15]

While educational requirements were very different for the three types of practitioners, they nonetheless tended to duplicate each other's efforts in the field, and although

---

[13] Miles, *Edinburgh School,* pp. 195, 208; Youngson, *Scientific Revolution,* p. 31.
[14] M. Jeanne Peterson, *The Medical Profession in Mid-Victorian London* (Berkeley: University of California Press, 1978), pp. 5–6, 8, 10–11, 17.
[15] Frederick F. Cartwright, *The Development of Modern Surgery* (London: Arthur Barker Limited, 1967), p. 17.

the three professions continually asserted their uniqueness, the reality of nineteenth-century medical practice made it difficult to maintain these traditional divisions.[16]

The transformations brought about by industrialization increasingly widened the gap between the official, lawful position of the three professions and what was actually done by their respective members. In practice physicians did more than advise and prescribe, surgeons diagnosed internal maladies, and by 1848 most apothecaries doubled as surgeons. Parliament attempted to remedy this situation by passing the Medical Act of 1858, establishing the General Council of Medical Education and Registration which supervised the training and commissioning of practitioners throughout the British Isles. The act stipulated that all who were qualified to practice medicine register with the Council, and a yearly list of their names was published.[17]

Not surprisingly, students of medical history agree that surgeons did not perform many invasive operations in the first half of the 1800s, especially before the use of anesthetics. The two most obvious reasons for so few of these surgeries being done were the unbearable pain and the unacceptably high death rate they caused. Even after the introduction of chloroform, which afforded surgeons more time to perfect their art, one-third of all amputees died. Indeed, the use of chloroform contributed to an increase in the overall number of fatalities because surgeons became more willing to use the knife in spite of the fact that infections remained as prevalent as ever.[18]

In 1853 the Glasgow Royal Infirmary published a report containing an analysis of 284 amputations performed during a recent ten-year period. It showed that the chances of dying from amputations were as follows: for the forearm, one in six; for the arm, two in three; for the leg, even odds; and for the thigh, two to one. Based on this record it is easy to understand why one observer noted that "patients, no matter how critical their need, dread the very name of hospital, and the most skilful surgeons distrust their own craft."[19]

Guy Williams, a country practitioner's son who was named for the founder of the famous Guy's Hospital in London, captured the essence of early nineteenth-century popular attitudes toward hospitals when he declared, "No sick or injured person who could possibly be nursed at home or in a medical man's private residence would choose, in preference, to enter the squalid and crowded wards of the public institutions." Williams also claimed that hospital administrators considered fifty to sixty patients per ward to be "sound and economical hospital management," even though "many, if not the majority, of the patients would have come from the filthy and cholera-ridden slums that abounded at the time, and would have been chronically dirty." The lack of faith in institutions like these is understandable and may explain why the number of operations did not increase in Glasgow after anesthetics became available. The population of Scotland's largest city swelled, and the number of acci-

[16] Ivan Waddington, *The Medical Profession in the Industrial Revolution* (Dublin: Gill and Macmillan Humanities Press, 1984), pp. 47–48.

[17] Ivan Waddington, "General Practitioners and Consultants in Early Nineteenth-Century England: The Sociology of an Intra-Professional Conflict," in *Health Care and Popular Medicine in Nineteenth Century England,* ed. John Woodward and David Richards (New York: Holmes & Meier Publishers, 1977), pp. 165–68; Peterson, *Medical Profession,* pp. 34–35.

[18] Cartwright, *Modern Surgery,* pp. 12–13; Douglas Guthrie, *From Witchcraft to Antisepsis: A Study in Antithesis* (Lawrence, Kansas: University of Kansas Press, 1955), p. 32.

[19] Archibald Young, "Lord Lister's Life and Work," *Janus* 31 (May 1927): 321–22.

dents from industry rose markedly, but from 1846, when ether was introduced, until the early 1860s there was no corresponding growth in the amount of surgeries performed.[20]

Another conceivable reason for the percentage of operations in Glasgow remaining constant after the advent of anesthetics was the fact that the death toll there was already one of the worst in the British Isles, and surgeons did not want to add to those statistics. Both the Glasgow Royal Infirmary and the one in Edinburgh had "distinctly higher" mortality rates than other health care institutions in Great Britain before the introduction of the antiseptic method. One historian has attributed this to the fact that "they admitted elderly terminal patients." It should also be noted that the voluntary infirmaries "admitted patients only on the recommendation of a subscriber to the hospital," and such an individual was not likely to jeopardize the reputation of the institution.[21]

Although the outcome of surgery remained as uncertain as always, surgeons continually sought to improve survival rates by inventing new methods and treatments. This was especially true of those who did amputations. Alexander Miles, who wrote the history of pre-Listerian surgery at the Edinburgh Royal Infirmary, stated that surgeons were so ashamed of their inability to preserve the lives of amputees that they

> sought to avoid the "opprobrium of surgery" by adopting measures less drastic than amputation. In place of removing the limb, attempts were made to excise the diseased parts, and so great was the success that attended excision for tuberculosis and other disorganising diseases of joints that the operation became an established surgical procedure. It is true that these operations did not eliminate the risk of sepsis, and they involved a long and often dangerous convalescence, but, if the patient survived, his limb had been conserved, even if it was not always sound and useful.[22]

Other surgeons resorted to simple procedures such as irrigating amputation wounds with cold water and leaving them open for a while before binding their edges with adhesives. Liston, who developed a transparent mucilage, employed a version of this technique that resulted in an 11.4 percent hospital death rate. One German surgeon even used vinegar dressings on open wounds, and his fatality rate for amputations was only six percent. By way of comparison, Lister's percentage of deaths from amputations was 11.25. All of these successes were impressive in light of the fact that before the use of antiseptics approximately forty percent of amputees died.[23]

---

[20] Guy Williams, *The Age of Miracles: Medicine and Surgery in the Nineteenth Century* (London: Constable, 1981), pp. 89–90; David Hamilton and Margaret Lamb, "Surgeons and surgery," in *Health Care as Social History: The Glasgow Case,* ed. Olive Checkland and Margaret Lamb (Aberdeen, Scotland: Aberdeen University Press, 1982), pp. 77–79.

[21] F. B. Smith, *The People's Health, 1830–1910* (New York: Holmes & Meier Publishers, Inc., 1979), p. 271; Carolyn I. Pennington, "Mortality and Medical Care in Nineteenth-Century Glasgow," *Medical History* 23 (October 1979): 444, 447.

[22] Alexander Miles, "Before the Dawn," in *Joseph, Baron Lister: Centenary Volume, 1827–1927,* ed. A. Logan Turner (Edinburgh: Oliver and Boyd, 1927), p. 32.

[23] Owen H. Wangensteen, Sarah D. Wangensteen, and Charles F. Klinger, "Some Pre-Listerian and Post-Listerian Antiseptic Wound Practices and the Emergence of Asepsis," *Surgery, Gynecology & Obstetrics* 137 (October 1973): 678; Gordon, *Disasters,* p. 19; Youngson, *Scientific Revolution,* p. 203.

The most innovative technique for dealing with wound sepsis, though, was one that evolved from the practice of Ignaz Semmelweis, an Hungarian obstetrician who introduced an ingeniously simple way to stop the spread of puerperal fever while he was serving as a physician's assistant in a maternity clinic at the Vienna General Hospital in 1847. He promoted the use of a chloride of lime solution, initially for the purpose of removing the scent of corpses from the hands of those who performed autopsies on patients who died in the clinic. This killed any decomposing substances that remained after routine cleansing. "In fact, Semmelweis was warning against *all* decaying organic matter—not just against a specific contagion that originated from victims of childbed fever itself."[24]

Regardless of how broadly Semmelweis conceived the danger from dead organic materials to be, his chief contribution to medical history was to markedly reduce mortality rates in the various clinics where he worked. He achieved this by merely washing his hands, after each of his bedside visits, with "a chlorine solution until the skin was slippery." Indeed, he was able to virtually eradicate puerperal fever in three different lying-in hospitals. The percentage of mothers who died from postnatal infection dropped from 18.3 to 1.2. Lister later said that he did not learn about this approach to combating the spread of disease until after 1883, the year he traveled to Budapest, even though he had also visited Vienna only nine years after it was instituted. The evidence of his truthfulness is that after he knew about Semmelweis's method he shifted his emphasis from curative to preventive antisepticism.[25] (See Figure 2.)

These imaginative efforts to improve surgical techniques and general hospital practices had negligible effect, however, because of the nature of standard procedures before antisepsis. Little concerned for personal or environmental cleanliness,

> surgeons and dressers upon entering the wards removed their coats and donned some old and soiled one, respected for its years of service. In the buttonholes of these coats were usually several silk threads or ligatures ready to the hand, after an application of beeswax, whenever a stitch was needed. One or two jugs of water were ready in which to rinse the instruments or marine sponges as the surgeon went from bed to bed doing his dressings. Naturally, under these conditions no wounds were clean, and pus formation was so universal that it was considered a necessary part of the healing process.[26]

Nearly all surgery was done in hospitals, and conditions in them were usually deplorable. Public facilities were insufficiently lighted, poorly ventilated, unprofessionally administered, and overpopulated. Patients with communicable diseases were routinely placed in the same wards as those who suffered from such common complaints as broken bones.[27]

---

[24] K. Codell Carter and Barbara R. Carter, *Childbed Fever: A Scientific Biography of Ignaz Semmelweis* (Westport, Connecticut: Greenwood Press, 1994), pp. 44–45, 52–53, 56.

[25] Ibid., p. 69; Owen H. Wangensteen and Sarah D. Wangensteen, "Lister, His Books, and Evolvement of His Antiseptic Wound Practices," *Bulletin of the History of Medicine* 48 (Spring 1974): 121–22, 126–27; Nuland, *Doctors*, pp. 247, 358.

[26] Samuel W. Lambert and George M. Goodwin, *Medical Leaders from Hippocrates to Osler* (Indianapolis: The Bobbs-Merrill Company, 1929), p. 278.

[27] Ibid., pp. 277–78; Youngson, *Scientific Revolution*, pp. 23–24.

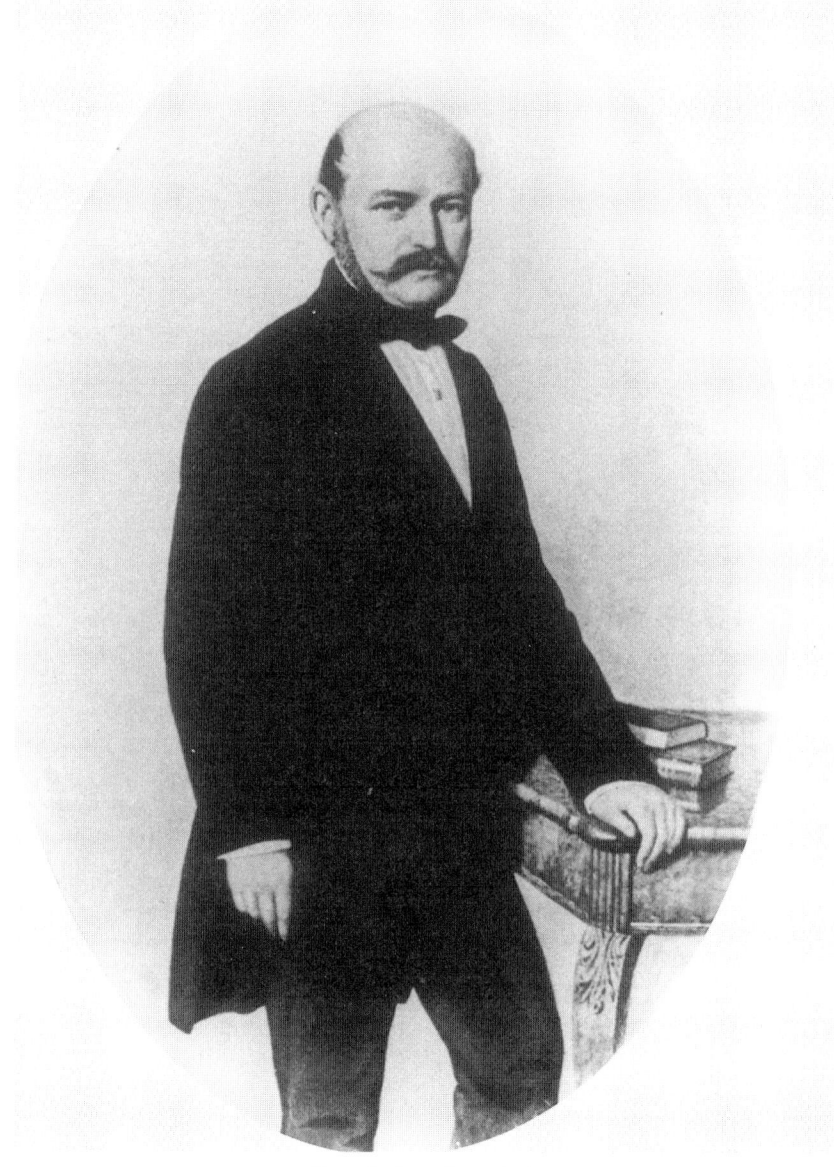

Figure 2. Ignaz Semmelweis

Conditions in surgical wards were worse than in the medical wards of hospitals. As F. B. Smith noted in his study of nineteenth-century British public health:

Operating-tables and rooms were not washed between operations: the wooden or linoleum-covered floor was simply sprinkled with sawdust. Into the 1870s at least, the wooden table was covered with a permanent, thick woollen red cloth, to absorb the blood. Some large hospitals had two tables in the one room: operations proceeded simultaneously. It was usual, too, until into the 1870s, to re-use bandages and sponges after they had been 'washed'. They were not boiled.[28]

Soiled dressings were indeed cleaned as soon as an operation was finished, and beds were aired when patients perished. However, surgical tools overlaid with rust-free materials were not substituted for iron implements until the 1870s. Additionally, hospital employees were not very well paid, and thus tended to be lax. Prior to 1860, when Florence Nightingale established a nursing school at London's St. Thomas Hospital, personnel usually came from lower class ranks and were "uneducated, unskilled, poor, slovenly, and often more interested in alcohol than in their patients." Patients were supposed to do certain things for themselves, though, like getting out of bed and eating. Their reward was a complete meal, including alcohol.[29]

Although military hospitals reflected their civilian counterparts, battlefield conditions made them even worse. The Crimean War was Europe's first major war since the fall of Napoleon, and the appalling state of medical care during it became known through the efforts of Florence Nightingale. She rose to prominence due to the care she gave wounded British soldiers in the Turkish town of Scutari, not far from Constantinople. A large barracks and hospital there had been commandeered by the army, but "cholera cases and battle casualties were crammed in together. There were no beds, no kitchens, no usable latrines." The amount of dirt present was staggering, and Nightingale claimed that there were more than a thousand troops suffering from diarrhea at the same time. Because of her work and that of thirty-eight fellow nurses who accompanied her the fatality rate fell from forty-two percent in January, 1855, to two percent six months later. This was in spite of "hostile and suspicious British doctors" who paid no attention to them. Nightingale was determined, however, then and for the remainder of her life, to provide both better training for nurses and treatment for patients. In the process she accumulated a wealth of evidence concerning epidemic diseases and has been called the "midwife to epidemiology."[30]

After the Crimean War Nightingale led a reform movement to improve hygienic conditions in the British armed forces. Her popularity, combined with public outrage over the conduct of the war's medical affairs, prompted the government to create the Army Sanitary Commission in 1857. The commission received extensive authority in matters pertaining to the sanitary condition of the home army, including the oversight of the Army Medical Department. Determined to go even further, however, Nightingale also targeted the colonial army in the wake of the Indian Mutiny. The result was the establishment of the Indian Sanitary Commission in 1859.

By 1859 Nightingale had formed definite opinions on hospital administration, which she expressed in her adroit *Notes on Hospitals*. The book addressed not only sanitation but also hospital construction and ward organization. It was well-received, and though "her views on ward ventilation and her commitment to the sprawling

---

[28] Smith, *People's Health,* pp. 267–68.
[29] Ibid., pp. 269–70; Youngson, *Scientific Revolution,* pp. 23–24.
[30] John P. Dolan and William N. Adams-Smith, *Health and Society: A Documentary History of Medicine* (New York: The Seabury Press, 1978), p. 153; Richard M. Krause, *The Restless Tide: The Persistent Challenge of the Microbial World* (Washington, D.C.: The National Foundation for Infectious Diseases, 1981), pp. 60–61, 64.

pavilion design were extreme, they were within the mainstream of British opinion at the time."[31] Nightingale began her description of how hospitals should be constructed by stating that the sick should be housed in separate pavilions, and she defined a pavilion as "a detached block of building." She went on to say that no block should have more than two floors of wards and that for each single pavilion there should only be one ward per floor. Next, Nightingale set the limit of patients for each ward at between twenty and thirty-two and contended that each bed should be allotted fifteen hundred cubic feet. This required that the height of each ward be no more than fifteen feet, the width approximately twenty-five feet, and the length eighty feet. Finally, she specified that there should be at least one window for every two beds.[32]

The medical profession was not noticeably affected by Nightingale's opinions until the third edition of her book appeared in 1863. This larger, more detailed issue included a table prepared by William Farr, the superintendent of the General Register Office's Statistical Department who was also one of the most important figures in nineteenth-century epidemiology. Based on registration and census data from two years earlier, the table compared mortality rates for 106 English hospitals and averaged them according to location. Nightingale accepted these figures as typical of normal populations and applicable to all health care institutions. The numbers revealed that the percentage of those who died was far greater in urban than in rural areas. Hospitals in London and other large cities had mortality rates more than twice as high as county or provincial institutions. Nightingale's interpretation of Farr's statistics infuriated the London medical establishment because she unequivocally asserted that "the most unhealthy hospitals" were in the metropolitan area, while "by far the most healthy" were in "the smaller country towns." The anger of the profession was directed at Farr, however, because Nightingale was too publicly admired and politically influential for her intentions or qualifications to be challenged outright.[33]

Supporters of hospitals did confront Nightingale's charges indirectly, though, by publicizing the percentages of patients cured in them. Thus, considerable disagreement followed concerning the extent to which people were or were not being healed. In the 1860s the dispute centered on what constituted a cure. Holistic approaches to illnesses were increasingly employed instead of simply trying to eradicate their physical manifestations. The alleviation of pain was the desired result, whether or not there was a corresponding return to health. By using such rationalizations, those who extolled the virtues of hospitals were able to claim great success in curing the sick without implementing the changes suggested by Nightingale.[34]

Nightingale, on the other hand, did not believe that hospitals cured people. Only nature could accomplish that. Hospitals and their staffs could facilitate the healing role of nature by impeding the spread of infection and equipping patients to resist it. Medicine, in Nightingale's view, did not play a crucial role in "the curative process."

---

[31] John M. Eyler, *Victorian Social Medicine: The Ideas and Methods of William Farr* (Baltimore: The Johns Hopkins University Press, 1979), pp. 159, 161–62, 172–73, 176, 178.

[32] Florence Nightingale, *Notes on Hospitals,* 3d ed. (London: Longman, Green, Longman, Roberts, and Green, 1863), pp. 56–67.

[33] David E. Lilienfeld, "'The Greening of Epidemiology': Sanitary Physicians and the London Epidemiological Society (1830–1870)," *Bulletin of the History of Medicine* 52 (Winter 1978): 507; Eyler, *Social Medicine,* pp. 9, 180–81.

[34] Smith, *People's Health,* pp. 265–68.

She never accepted the idea that specific microorganisms caused specific diseases and as late as 1893 referred to the use of disinfectants and antiseptics as "mystic rites." She did think that air played the most important part in the spread of diseases and even equated the actions of fermentation and putrefaction. A lack of cleanliness, though, produced illness. "She had seen filth produce remitting fever in a particular ward, a greater accumulation of filth change prevailing symptoms to those of typhoid, and, finally, still more dirt aggravate these symptoms into those of typhus."[35]

Renovations to hospitals were admittedly quite costly, especially to Nightingale's specifications, and they disrupted the day-to-day activities of medical personnel. Furthermore, since surgeons spent relatively little time in hospitals and those who died in them were not subject to coroners' inquests, it was easy for their managers to overlook sanitary concerns. This did not mean that surgeons were uninterested in public health. On the contrary, they were particularly distressed by the state of medical care because they lived "in a period when their inability to cure disease made it imperative to prevent it." Even Nightingale recognized that the nursing profession would be a dangerous occupation if there were no defenses against contagious diseases, though she thought security was gained through "prudence, proper regimen, and good general health."[36]

M. W. Flinn, in his introduction to *Report on the Sanitary Condition of the Labouring Population of Great Britain,* a ground-breaking study of Victorian public health conducted in the 1840s, offered an explanation for the nineteenth-century medical profession's interest in sanitary measures. Referring to "the springs of their passionate advocacy of a cleaner and healthier Britain," he noted the fact that most of them were trained at the University of Edinburgh and were taught to deal with health care issues within the context of a patient's social environment. Identifying a problem and solving it are two very different things, however, and most surgeons merely voiced their concerns to administrators as opposed to correcting matters themselves.[37]

Some hospital managers saw the need for improvements and listened to their staff members. The Glasgow Royal Infirmary built a new surgical wing the year that Nightingale's views on hospital construction were first published. It increased the number of beds to 200 and, with its high ceilings and broad wards, testified to the hospital's commitment to combat surgical mortality by increasing ventilation.[38] The infirmary's managers were determined to make their new building "the last word in hospital construction." All of the wards

> had thirty-five apertures for the admission of fresh air, not including doors. Six openings in the ceilings communicated with corresponding openings in the outer walls, three on each side of the ward, carried in channels between the joists. Fresh air was also admitted by screened windows, and fanlights above the ward doors.

---

[35] Charles E. Rosenberg, *Explaining Epidemics and Other Studies in the History of Medicine* (Cambridge: Cambridge University Press, 1992), pp. 92–93, 100, 103–105.

[36] Ibid., p. 104; Steven J. Novak, "Professionalism and Bureaucracy: English Doctors and the Victorian Public Health Administration," *Journal of Social History* 6 (Summer 1973): 443; Smith, *People's Health,* pp. 265–68.

[37] Edwin Chadwick, *Report of the Sanitary Condition of the Labouring Population of Great Britain,* ed. M. W. Flinn (Edinburgh: Edinburgh University Press, 1965), pp. 21–22; Smith, *People's Health,* pp. 265–68.

[38] Hamilton and Lamb, "Surgeons and surgery," pp. 77–79.

Separate ventilation was established for the sculleries, bath-rooms, and water-closets. In the basement "were the nurses' dormitories, store-rooms, and other necessary purposes." The report adds that "a large and commodious hoist has been erected, by means of which patients may be conveyed to the different floors."[39]

This detailed description provides the reader with a rare glimpse into the setting of Lister's antiseptic experiments which began in those same wards six years later.

A final issue, which due to government regulation affected the development of surgery in nineteenth-century Britain, was the antivivisection controversy. In 1876 Parliament passed the Cruelty to Animals Act on the urging of Prime Minister Benjamin Disraeli. The law reflected public sentiment that had kept medical research in Great Britain from attaining the level reached on the Continent, although it did not prohibit the vivisection of animals without backbones and permitted licensed experimentation with cats and dogs.[40]

Queen Victoria supported the legislation and had even asked Lister in 1875 to speak out against vivisection. He had successfully lanced an abscess under her left arm four years earlier, but because he occasionally engaged in the dissection of living animals himself and because of the importance of the practice to medical science he refused to honor the Queen's wishes. Lister did, however, send her a letter stating his belief that vivisection should always be done with anesthetics but added that the hunting of animals for amusement, unkind methods for disciplining them, and unnatural ways of reproducing and fattening them were crueler than the tests performed on them in laboratories. Indeed, part of the explanation for the inertia which Lister encountered among British surgeons lies in their negative attitude toward vivisection, an outlook that was peculiar to the 1800s because such medical pioneers as William Harvey and Edward Jenner had experimented with live animals.[41]

In 1824, though, only one year after Jenner's death, the Society for the Prevention of Cruelty to Animals was founded. It adopted a platform which roundly indicted all pain inflicted by vivisectors based on the principle "that Providence cannot intend that the secrets of Nature should be discovered by means of cruelty." Conversely, it also recognized the need for certain crucial tests "under the control of a benevolent mind."[42] This compromised the group's moral and ethical standards because it was in the days before anesthesia, when no experimentation could be carried out without suffering.

After gaining royal status in 1840, the organization gradually became more political and by 1857 was determined to "begin active involvement in the practical problems of the control of vivisection." The latter year is when news of the dissection of

---

[39] James A. Morris, "The Royal Infirmary Buildings," in *Lister & the Lister Ward* (Glasgow: Jackson, Wylie and Co., 1927), pp. 41, 43.
[40] Mark N. Ozer, "The British Vivisection Controversy," *Bulletin of the History of Medicine* 40 (March-April 1966): 166–67.
[41] Cuthbert Dukes, *Lord Lister (1827–1912)* (London: Leonard Parsons, 1924), pp. 146–47, 152–53; Ira S. Goldenberg, "Joseph Lister: Innovation and Insurgency in Surgery," *Connecticut Medicine* 40 (November 1976): 772.
[42] Quoted in Richard D. French, *Antivivisection and Medical Science in Victorian Society* (Princeton, New Jersey: Princeton University Press, 1975), pp. 27–28.

living horses by French veterinarians to improve their surgical skills reached the members, and they formed a committee to discuss the matter with Napoleon III. The emperor did meet with representatives from the society but not until April, 1861, and no consistent policy was ever formulated for France. In August of the following year an international congress met at the Crystal Palace to discuss the controversy, and the English delegates finally agreed "that vivisection under anesthesia was permissible, since without pain there could be no cruelty."[43]

Once a consensus was reached, the medical journals of Great Britain disseminated majority opinions concerning when experimentation on living animals was unacceptable. For the purpose of acquiring surgical expertise, it was vehemently denounced, and as a method for classroom instruction it was explicitly discouraged. Lister, one of the few British surgeons who practiced vivisection, perceived that a more serious problem lay with those opposed to it, agreeing with vivisectionists that the antivivisection movement stood in the way of physiological research and the advancement of biomedical science.[44] He stated that those who opposed experiments on living animals had good intentions but that their deeds were "based upon ignorance." Elaborating on their lack of understanding, he added, "They allow that man is permitted to inflict pain upon the lower animals, when some substantial advantage is to be gained; but they deny that any good has ever resulted from the researches which they condemn." This glaring inconsistency of antivivisectionists frustrated Lister, but he continued to refer to the impact of previous vivisections in arguing that "from the discovery of the circulation of the blood onwards, our knowledge of healthy animal function has been mainly derived from experiments on animals."[45]

Therefore, when Lister set out in 1867 to challenge his brotherhood to employ a new technique for conquering hospital diseases, he encountered numerous professional, institutional, and political obstacles along the way. In order for surgeons to be able to stop the massive loss of life in British health care institutions, something had to be done to overcome regional differences in medical education so that all university-trained practitioners could receive firsthand experience with the human body. Also, the regimentation of the medical profession needed to be relaxed in order for there to be greater cooperation between the members of the different fields. Any resistance to improvements in hospital construction had to be met by a united front of politically active medical men. The refusal of some surgeons to consider innovative methods should be summarily condemned in the hope of jolting the profession out of its complacency. Finally, progress demanded that the restrictiveness of the antivivisection movement be ignored.

---

[43] Ibid., pp. 30–32; Ozer, "Vivisection Controversy," p. 160.
[44] French, *Antivivisection,* p. 33; Nicolaas A. Rupke, "Pro-vivisection in England in the Early 1880s: Arguments and Motives," in *Vivisection in Historical Perspective,* ed. Nicolaas A. Rupke (London: Croom Helm, 1987), pp. 197–98.
[45] Stephen Paget, *Experiments on Animals,* with an Introduction by Lord Lister (New York: William Wood & Company, 1900), pp. xi–xii.

2. Social Interpretation as a Factor in the Diffusion of Listerism

Before Lister emerged on the medical scene in Great Britain, two divergent social theories existed regarding the spread of disease: contagionism and anticontagionism. Supporters of contagionism speculated that disease was caused by the transmission of a physical or chemical property from one person to another through bodily contact or from the air, assuming the distance was not too far. That belief dated from the sixteenth century but had never been tested scientifically, and nineteenth-century liberals associated it with excessive bureaucratic regimentation because it was used to justify quarantines which hindered free trade. Those who wanted to be rational in their approach to medicine in the 1800s viewed contagionism as the last vestige of medieval mysticism. They wanted to limit government interference in the private sector and saw contagionists as disguised mercantilists. Anticontagionists, therefore, tended to be mostly scientists and reformers who championed the rights of the individual against reactionary measures by the authorities. They subscribed to a miasmatic theory to explain illnesses, blaming bad smells and filth as the causes of disease. Miasma were specifically defined by anticontagionists as "poison arising from decaying animal or vegetable matter." Thus, they endeavored to solve the social problems of industrial Great Britain through waste removal, convinced that the answer to disease prevention was cleanliness.[1]

Cholera was the most difficult disease for contagionists to explain because it clearly did not afflict all who came into contact with it and because it was most severe where miasma were. When the first outbreak of cholera occurred in England in 1831, most physicians were still contagionists, but by the time the second epidemic had run its course in 1849, the opposite was true. To rationalize cholera's selectivity, some who had been pure contagionists revised their theory to allow for "contingent" or "modified" contagionism. Ultimately, though, during the eighteen-year interim most became strict anticontagionists.[2] The explanation of anticontagionists for the cause of cholera, however, was no better than that of their adversaries. They termed its origin "doubtful" and simply labeled it a non-contagious epidemic. Then they conveniently stipulated that non-contagious diseases could never become contagious. They believed that the cause of the disease was spontaneously generated, but offered no answer to the question of why only selected areas were affected.[3] Both sides recognized that being exposed to contagion or miasma did not necessarily mean that one would become sick, and both listed what they looked upon as the predisposing causes of the illness. The most complete enumeration appeared in *The Lancet,* England's leading medical

---

[1] David L. Cowen, "Liberty, Laissez-Faire and Licensure in Nineteenth Century Britain," *Bulletin of the History of Medicine* 43 (January–February 1969): 30; Erwin H. Ackerknecht, "Anticontagionism between 1821 and 1867," *Bulletin of the History of Medicine* 22 (September-October 1948): 565–68.
[2] Ackerknecht, "Anticontagionism," pp. 576, 578.
[3] Margaret Pelling, *Cholera, Fever and English Medicine, 1825–1865* (Oxford: Oxford University Press, 1978), pp. 22–25.

journal, in November, 1831. It attributed cholera to "crowded population, poverty, filth, foul air, unwholesome food, especially bad water, depressing passions, habits of intemperance, defective clothing, and general bodily debility."[4]

Cholera was particularly shocking because of the suddenness with which it struck and the rapidity with which it spread. Many hundreds of thousands became ill, and tens of thousands died. Also, the middle and upper classes were more likely to succumb to it because it was a water-borne disease and they had greater access to water. Since they administered the cities and counties, they immediately commissioned local governmental agencies to look into the problem.[5] Another reason cholera was so feared was that those who contracted it occasionally died in a matter of hours after the symptoms of the disease began to manifest themselves. More often, it took several days for one to die. An especially morbid aspect of cholera was the fact that some who had it looked as if they were dead before they actually were, and seemingly everyone had heard of cases where prematurely buried sufferers tried "to claw free of the coffin." Rumors also persisted that medical students were using cholera victims for anatomy practice and that they did not always wait for the victims to die naturally. Of even more immediate concern, though, were the reports of presumably healthy people suddenly perishing from the disease.[6]

The symptoms of cholera were indeed striking and horrible. The body grew cold, the pulse could not be heard, and frequently victims could do no more than lie prostrate. Also, the disease was accompanied by "two or three days of a diarrhea which increased in intensity and became accompanied by a painful retching; thirst and dehydration; severe pain in the limbs, stomach, and abdominal muscles; a change in skin hue to a sort of bluish gray."[7] William Gairdner, professor of medicine at Glasgow during the time that Lister was there, penned a book entitled *Public Health in Relation to Air and Water* in which he poignantly assessed the horror cholera engendered as compared to the other epidemics that Britons had encountered. With a very florid style he reflected,

> Our other plagues were home-bred, and part of ourselves, as it were; we had a habit of looking on them with a fatal indifference, indeed, inasmuch as it led us to believe that they could be effectually subdued. But the cholera was something outlandish, unknown, monstrous [*sic*]; its tremendous ravages, so long foreseen and feared, so little to be explained, its insidious march over whole continents, its apparent defiance of all the known and conventional precautions against the spread of epidemic disease, invested it with a mystery and a terror which thoroughly took hold of the public mind, and seemed to recall the memory of the great epidemics of the middle ages.[8]

---

[4] Quoted in R. J. Morris, *Cholera, 1832: The Social Response to an Epidemic* (New York: Holmes & Meier Publishers, 1976), p. 174.

[5] Edwin Chadwick, *Report on the Sanitary Condition of the Labouring Population of Great Britain*, ed. M. W. Flinn (Edinburgh: Edinburgh University Press, 1965), pp. 8, 10.

[6] Anthony S. Wohl, *Endangered Lives: Public Health in Victorian Britain* (Cambridge, Massachusetts: Harvard University Press, 1983), pp. 118–19.

[7] Ibid; Bruce Haley, *The Healthy Body and Victorian Culture* (Cambridge, Massachusetts: Harvard University Press, 1978), p. 6.

[8] Quoted in Haley, *Healthy Body,* p. 6.

Cholera first appeared in Britain in October, 1831, and by 1833 approximately 23,000 people were dead. The second and worst appearance of the disease occurred in 1848–49 when 53,000 died. The third outbreak, in 1853–54, also caused 23,000 deaths. The fourth and final appearance of the disease, in 1866, only killed 14,000 because enough was known about it by then to provide some safeguards.[9] Contributing to the terror accompanying the first epidemic was the fact that there was no consensus of opinion on how to approach the problem. The medical establishment could not agree on a theory that explained the origin of cholera and therefore gave the public conflicting advice on the best means for preventing the spread of the disease. Contagionists offered one kind of advice; anticontagionists offered another that was diametrically opposed. Moreover, neither one could provide a completely satisfactory explanation for the disease's progress. Indeed, they differed so greatly that even agreement on terminology and a conceptual framework for discussion was impossible.[10]

All epidemic diseases were capable of providing evidence that could be used to support either the contagionist or the anticontagionist view, but cholera was especially vexing. Contagionists could show how cholera had followed lines of human communication as it spread from the Indian subcontinent. It clearly had followed routes favored by traders, armies, and pilgrims. Contagionists could also refute the miasmatic interpretation by stressing that bad smells did not always cause disease and that during the winter, when they were less noticeable, many diseases were more common than in the summer. On the other hand, anticontagionists could point to the fact that cholera did not spread gradually or continuously. It did not always strike entire households at the same time, it could devastate one region while sparing another, and it could jump hundreds of miles.[11]

The first instance of cholera in the United Kingdom showed how puzzling the disease was, and indeed, shocked many in the medical profession who had come to accept the contagionist argument. Contagionists were astonished when physicians and nurses working with cholera victims were not stricken with the disease, as they often were during typhus epidemics. Also, the affliction struck hardest in "low-lying, densely populated, filthy areas." To explain such evidence contagionists argued that the more people there were in a given area, the more likely it was that the infection rate would increase. They also stressed that one should not assume contact with the disease had not been made just because a personal link could not be established. However, they were quick to point out that overcrowded, dirty dwellings were not the cause, since those conditions had existed previous to the occurrence of the epidemic. In their minds such houses were breeding grounds for cholera when it came but not the source of it.

Miasmatists believed that people living in filth were predisposed to infection and looked for susceptibility in factors like human behavior, humidity, and atmospheric electricity.[12] They also thought that the argument used by contagionists was mere sophistry. It was difficult, after all, to dispute maps of cholera outbreaks which showed

[9] Pelling, *Cholera*, p. 2.
[10] Morris, *Cholera, 1832*, p. 176.
[11] Ibid., pp. 177–79; Chadwick, *Sanitary Condition*, p. 63.
[12] Morris, *Cholera, 1832*, pp. 179–80.

that instances of the disease almost perfectly coincided with quarters that were indeed low-lying and unclean. Consequently, by 1848 when the second and most destructive cholera epidemic began, anticontagionism had come to dominate official thinking. The theory had also found a master propagandist in Edwin Chadwick, the secretary of the newly created General Board of Health which had been established by the Public Health Act of 1848. Like Chadwick, the Board was "aggressively miasmatic."[13]

Though cholera was the most frightening ailment of the 1800s, it was not the most devastating. One of the numerous students of this illness has placed it in proper perspective relative to other maladies. "As a cause of death and debility in mid-nineteenth-century England," she argues,

> cholera was surpassed among epidemic diseases by 'common continued fever' (chiefly typhoid, relapsing fever, and some typhus), scarlet fever, smallpox, and measles, and accounted for only a very small proportion of the area of highest mortality, which occurred among infants and young children. All the known epidemic diseases were exceeded in incidence and effect by the many forms of tuberculosis, the different appearances of which were regarded, until about the middle of the century, as distinct diseases and as being constitutional, not epidemic.[14]

Also, in terms of getting legislation passed, the greatest impetus for sanitary reform in England was not the initial occurrence of cholera but Edwin Chadwick's *Report on the Sanitary Condition of the Labouring Population of Great Britain* which can be viewed as the high water mark of anticontagionism in the United Kingdom. Chadwick was Secretary to the Poor Law Commission when his bluebook was published in 1842, and it is safe to say that by then the vast majority of medical practitioners agreed with it. His study was based on the findings of approximately one thousand Medical Officers of Health, who had been hired by the national government to enforce the Poor Law of 1834. Chadwick singled out journeymen tailors as a group of workers noted for their early deaths and attributed those deaths to poor ventilation and overcrowding. Then, he advocated prevention of disease through improvements in those two conditions at the workplace and in the private dwellings of the workers. His recommendation was based on the practicality of the situation because it was more cost-effective to correct the problems which caused sickness beforehand than to relieve suffering after the onset of disease.[15]

Chadwick also wrote a great deal about the importance of good drains, attributing illnesses such as rheumatism to "damp and marsh miasma from the want of drainage." He argued that fevers were due to "the air from neglected privies, and the miasma from the wet and undrained court or street." On diseases that were epidemic or endemic, he hedged somewhat by arguing that they were "caused, or aggravated, or propagated . . . by atmospheric impurities produced by decomposing animal and vegetable substances." If he was unsure about what caused diseases like cholera, he was certain that more people had died from filth than from wars.[16]

---

[13] Ibid., pp. 183–84, 202, 204–05; Ackerknecht, "Anticontagionism," pp. 567, 578–79.
[14] Pelling, *Cholera*, pp. 3–4, 6.
[15] Chadwick, *Sanitary Condition*, pp. 45, 47, 167, 173.
[16] Ibid., pp. 196–97; Wohl, *Endangered Lives*, p. 147.

Although contagionists were in the minority when Chadwick's book appeared, they also had powerful spokesmen. Foremost among these were John Snow and William Budd. Snow was a prestigious surgeon from London, whose published remarks on cholera first appeared in 1849 as the second epidemic of the disease came to an end. More importantly, four years later, after additional research, he surmised that cholera "always commences with disturbances of the functions of the alimentary canal; all the early symptoms are connected with this canal, and the effects which follow are only the results of what have occurred." Budd was a physician from Bristol who focused mainly on typhoid, a disease which was endemic in urban areas during the nineteenth century. Though typhoid was his specialty, Budd also postulated that cholera was caused by "a living organism of a distinct species, which was taken by the act of swallowing it, which multiplied in the intestine by self propagation."[17]

As early as 1839 Budd had conjectured, in an essay entitled "On the Causes and Mode of Propagation of the Common Continued Fevers of Great Britain and Ireland," that typhoid was caused by a different species than other fevers, and this undoubtedly influenced his thinking concerning the cause of cholera as well. He was not equivocal, however, in his assertion that typhoid was communicated and propagated by contagion.[18] A decade after writing his essay, Budd sent a letter to *The Lancet* in which he referred to "living organisms" in the intestines as the cause of cholera, describing them as "peculiar to a single species." For lack of a better word, he called them "fungi" and included them in the category of parasites. He also explained that they did not feed on waste products in the intestines but on "the constituents of the perfect blood." Consequently, he concluded that they could not "have been reared" in the intestines, but must have entered the body from an external source.[19]

Even though Budd was close to discovering the cause of cholera, it was the second edition of Snow's *On the Mode of Communication of Cholera,* published in 1855, that decisively refuted miasmatic explanations of the disease. This edition was much larger than the first one in 1849, which Snow himself said "was only a slender pamphlet." What made his second study of the subject so conclusive was the direct correlation he established between polluted water and the spread of cholera. He provided proof that in order to contract cholera polluted water or "minute quantities of the ejections and dejections of cholera patients must be swallowed." Physicians and nurses did not usually become ill after treating cholera patients because of the brevity of their visits and the fact that family members generally cleaned up the "ejections and dejections" of their loved ones. Also, those who did autopsies on the victims of cholera washed their hands afterwards. In addition to the evidence he presented to establish the cause of cholera, Snow expressed his opinion that other diseases like the plague, yellow fever, and typhoid were probably spread the same way.[20] (See Figure 3.)

Knowing that cholera was passed on by other means than water, Snow tactfully "assured his readers that accepting the water-borne theory of cholera implied preven-

---

[17] Quoted in Morris, *Cholera, 1832,* p. 207.
[18] William Budd, *On the Causes of Fevers (1839),* ed. Dale C. Smith (Baltimore: The Johns Hopkins University Press, 1984), pp. 47, 55.
[19] William Budd, "To the Editor of The Lancet," *The Lancet* (13 October 1849): 399.
[20] John Snow, *On the Mode of Communication of Cholera,* 2d ed. (London: John Churchill, 1855; reprint ed., New York: The Commonwealth Fund, 1936), pp. iii, v, 14–17, 125–29.

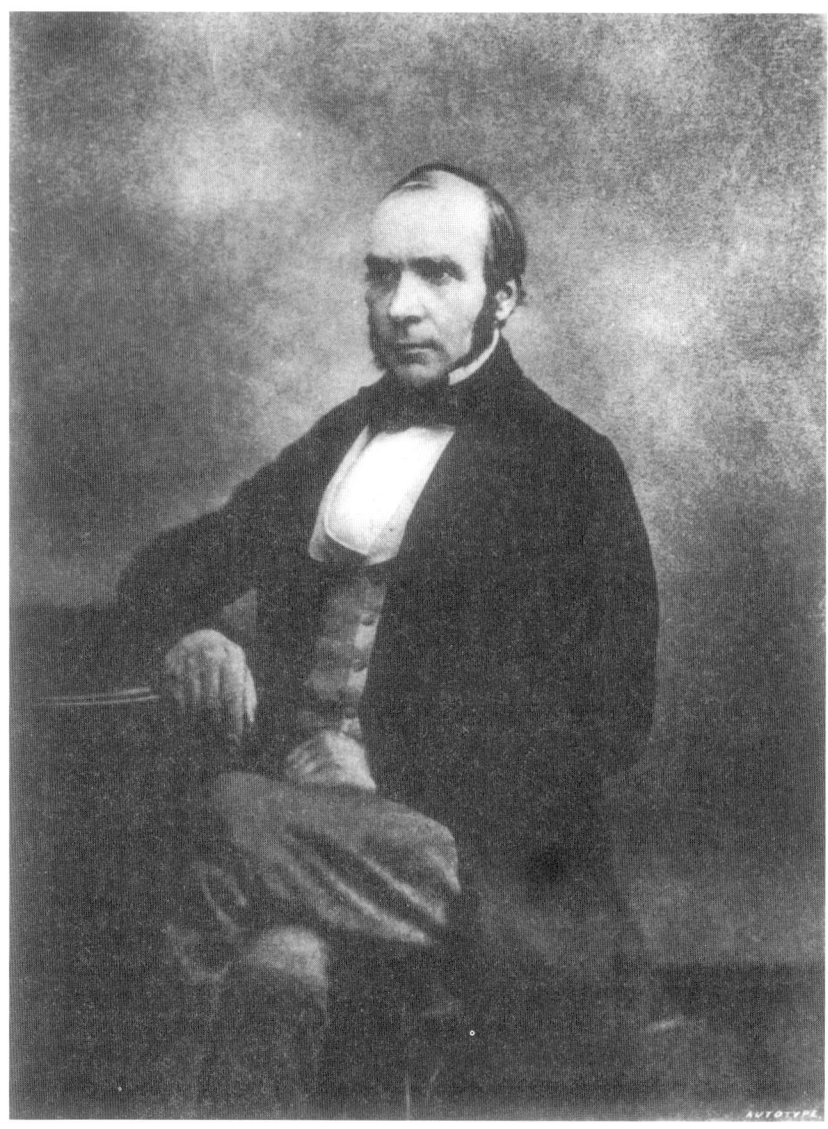

Figure 3. John Snow

tion by 'simple measures that will not interfere with social and commercial inter-course'." In effect Snow was assuring the economic community that the contagionist theory did not have to be at odds with liberal political and economic beliefs. It increas-ingly was, though, especially after 1866 when William Farr provided conclusive evi-dence for contagionism by tracing the last incidence of cholera to London's water supply. He found that open ponds of polluted water were being used to supply emer-gency drinking water, and when this practice ceased, the epidemic stopped. Laissez faire also ended because rulers "came to realize that these were national problems requiring solution on a national scale," even though they continued "paying lip-service to 'laissez-faire', the sanctity of individual effort and the deep-rooted rights of local government."[21]

Farr studied England's last three cholera epidemics, as well as smallpox and cattle plague, and "was the first person to adequately describe an epidemic numerically." He showed statistically how epidemics increase and decrease "in a predictable manner" and traced their spread geographically and topographically. He also coined the term "zymotic" to equate fermentation with the chemical changes "that occurred during the attack of an epidemic, endemic, or contagious disease." His report on the 1866 cholera outbreak "made the water-borne theory 'irresistible,'" according to *The Lancet*. It also "called attention to the importance of Pasteur's work on fermentation." Before the next decade passed, Farr "had accepted the major features of the germ theory."[22]

John Snow had expired unexpectedly in 1858, but he is "commonly regarded as a voice crying in the wilderness for the germ theory" which Pasteur had put before the scientific community a year earlier. In spite of Snow's contributions, it is important to note that his commitment to contagionism was really very limited and that he showed no great allegiance to the germ theory in his writings. Moreover, he freely acknowledged the probable role of spontaneous generation in diseases like erysipelas which cause putrefaction.[23] William Budd, on the other hand, not only supported the germ theory but also vigorously opposed both anticontagionism and spontaneous generation in his seminal work *Typhoid Fever: Its Nature, Mode of Spreading, and Prevention*, which was published in 1873.

Budd's book provided proof that typhoid was "a contagious or self-propagating fever," and he added, "It is scarcely to the credit of the medical profession that this great truth should still be disputed." He went on to express his belief that "the great majority, not of the laity only, but of the profession also, still remain anti-contagionists." Budd also admitted being perplexed and discouraged by the "direct opposition of opinion to fact in a matter of such vital importance, and so open to observation." He specifically held the General Board of Health accountable for much of the opposition he and other contagionists had faced. As he ended his book, Budd noted that just because the "germ of fever" in cases of typhoid could not be seen or traced, one should still not infer "that this fever ever does arise spontaneously." All should remember, Budd concluded, that his subject was a matter of "life or death to myriads of men," while other studies, like Darwin's theory of evolution, were "abstract only."[24]

Darwin's *Origin of Species* was published in 1859, and Budd was one of very few

---

[21] Morris, *Cholera, 1832*, pp. 209–10; John M. Eyler, "Mortality Statistics and Victorian Health Policy: Program and Criticism," *Bulletin of the History of Medicine* 50 (Fall 1976): 345; Ruth G. Hodgkinson, "Social Medicine and the Growth of Statistical Information," in *Medicine and Science in the 1860s*, ed. F. N. L. Poynter (London: Wellcome Institute for the History of Medicine, 1968), p. 184.

[22] John M. Eyler, *Victorian Social Medicine: The Ideas and Methods of William Farr* (Baltimore: The Johns Hopkins University Press, 1979), pp. 103, 106–107, 111–114, 119.

[23] Pelling, *Cholera*, pp. 203, 207, 213.

[24] William Budd, *Typhoid Fever: Its Nature, Mode of Spreading, and Prevention* (London: Longmans, Green, and Co., 1873), pp. 4–6, 8, 11, 180–81.

medical scientists who realized that the theory of evolution incidentally proposed "an account of the origin and distribution of disease and of the phenomenon of obligate parasitism." Though normally cautious in expressing opinions like the one on Darwinism, Budd could not resist labeling the bulk of physicians and all sanitarians as advocates of spontaneous generation. According to one astute observer, Darwin's book could have established a paradigm for judging the scientific merit of subsequent researches, but debates about its applicability hampered the full implementation of the evolutionary model, a circumstance which might have been avoided if "medical scientists had been more involved in the public debate on Darwinism in the 1860s." *The Lancet,* for example, made no mention of Darwin's book until 1866.[25] One year later, though, Listerism and the germ theory on which it was based provided medicine with a paradigm that proved to be totally relevant, producing a shift to a new model for healing.[26]

Budd penned some of his strongest words for the medical profession on the consequences of adhering to the theory of spontaneous generation in *The British Medical Journal,* the official publication of the British Medical Association. First of all, said Budd, "there is no proof whatever" that "the poisons of specific contagious diseases ever originate spontaneously." This meant that such diseases might eventually be prevented, but not until the medical community rejected the theory of spontaneous generation. Thus, as "long as opinion remains divided as to this cardinal point, it is vain to hope for the general adoption of any definite scheme of preventive measures."[27] Budd was more specific about the environmental factors that miasmatists were looking for to justify their position in his later definitive study of typhoid. He stated that "organic matter, and especially sewage in a state of decomposition, without any relation to antecedent fever, is still generally supposed to be the most fertile source."[28] (See Figure 4.)

Not all who adhered to the notion of spontaneous generation for explaining the origin of disease necessarily accepted the miasmatic interpretation for the spread of disease; the two should not be equated. Epidemics like those of cholera "instantly appeared and just as quickly disappeared. They claimed victims at random, regardless of age, race, class, or sex." Thus, the medical profession was prone to blame them on bad air. Other epidemics, like that of puerperal or childbed fever, produced "a 'grass roots' contagionist movement" due to the fact that they "could be traced because of the peculiar state of those exposed to its attack; that is, immobilized, pregnant women."[29]

Erwin H. Ackerknecht has identified the point at which there was a shift in the

---

[25] Pelling, *Cholera,* pp. 255, 263; Bernard Towers, "The Impact of Darwin's *Origin of Species* on Medicine and Biology," in *Medicine and Science in the 1860s,* ed. F. N. L. Poynter (London: Wellcome Institute for the History of Medicine, 1968), pp. 47–48, 50.

[26] For a classic discussion of paradigm shifts, which are as appropriate for understanding the history of medicine as they are other disciplines, see the seminal work, Thomas S. Kuhn, *The Structure of Scientific Revolutions* (Chicago: The University of Chicago Press, 1962), pp. 2–3, 7.

[27] William Budd, "Investigation of Epidemic and Epizootic Diseases," *The British Medical Journal* (24 September 1864): 356.

[28] Quoted in Haley, *Healthy Body,* p. 10.

[29] Gail Pat Parsons, "The British Medical Profession and Contagion Theory: Puerperal Fever as a Case Study, 1830–1860," *Medical History* 22 (April 1978): 149.

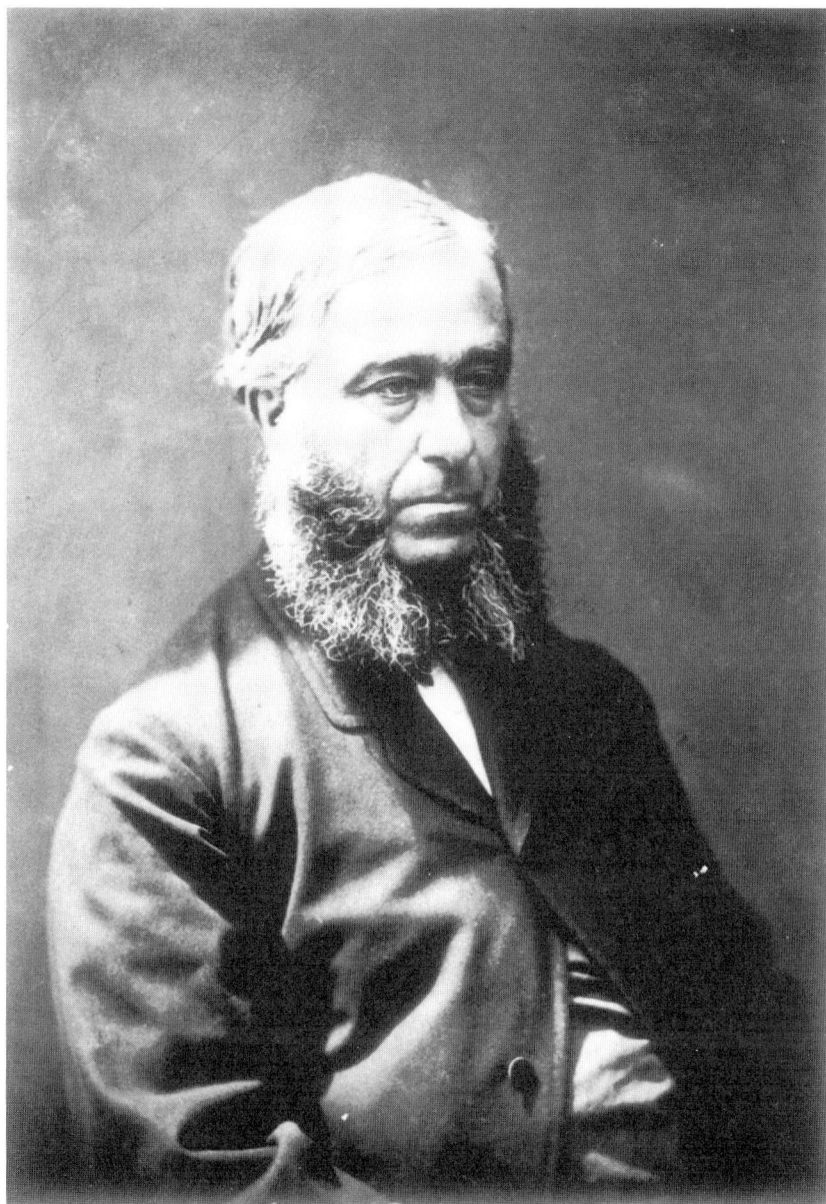

Figure 4. William Budd

attitudes of medical men from anticontagionism to contagionism. Elaborating on nineteenth-century cholera epidemics in general, he concluded that as a result of the third outbreak "and even more so during the fourth" that "the majority of the profession returned to contagion."[30] A perplexing paradox had faced anticontagionists in the period between the third and fourth episodes of cholera. A phenomenon known as the "Great Stink" occurred in 1858 and 1859. During these years the smell from sewage decaying in the Thames River could hardly be tolerated. It was particularly onerous in summertime, and inhabitants of London chose to go out of their way instead of using bridges and steamboats. Members of Parliament covered their windows, using material saturated with disinfectants, so that they could perform their responsibilities. Worst of all for miasmatists, an epidemic did not occur because of the smell, even though diseases such as typhoid were most serious in the heat of summer.[31]

Physicians were not the only ones to reconsider how diseases were spread. Vestrymen and other officials in cities like London began to behave in ways that showed they were no longer true believers in anticontagionism. In particular, they started concentrating more of their energies on projects designed to prevent human waste from coming into contact with water supplies. In St. Pancras, for example, fifteen miles of new sewers were installed between 1856 and 1870. Nine of the fifteen were laid by private companies, but the vestry supervised their work. The parish also built more drains, increasing the number of houses served by over seven thousand. In addition to these major projects, more than 20,000 minor tasks were performed by inspectors for the vestry. They filled cesspools and closed underground living areas used by the homeless. In private dwellings they installed cisterns and water closets, added dustbins, and removed farm animals. They inspected businesses such as bakehouses, slaughterhouses, and shelters for cattle. Last of all, they restricted occupations that were offensive to the public like melting tallow and cooking cats.

The legal justification for these measures was the Sanitary Act of 1866, which permitted authorities to control "overcrowding in houses let in lodgings or occupied by more than one family."[32] This was Great Britain's first major public health law, and it had been enacted because of the influence of miasmatists who had lobbied for the eradication of filth. Chadwick had endeavored to correct the problems of "inadequate sewerage and accumulations of excrement" because they produced what he referred to both as the "epidemic atmosphere" and as "deleteriously impregnated air." To adequately provide for waste "removal, was, however, a long-term proposition and the epidemics called for immediate action."[33]

Chadwick lost his position in 1854 and four years later the General Board of Health for which he worked was dismantled. This aided medical scientists in their quest for more control over epidemic diseases because Chadwick was replaced by John Simon "as the central figure in public health." Simon had been the medical officer for the General Board of Health and served in that same capacity for the Privy Council from 1858 to 1876. He was one of the men most responsible for the passage of the

[30] Ackerknecht, "Anticontagionism," p. 581.
[31] Haley, *Healthy Body,* p. 10.
[32] David Owen, *The Government of Victorian London, 1855–1889: The Metropolitan Board of Works, the Vestries, and the City Corporation* (Cambridge, Massachusetts: The Belknap Press of Harvard University Press, 1982), pp. 300–301.
[33] Wohl, *Endangered Lives,* p. 121.

Medical Act of 1858, and his plans called for a national organization supervised by a pathologist and staffed with medical experts. He had served as president of both the Pathological Society of London and the Royal College of Surgeons. Contrary to Simon, Chadwick had held physicians in "contempt" and "his greatest animus was reserved for medicine." Chadwick had looked upon their practices "as mere obstructions to the principles of health" and had not allowed them to sit on his board until it was required by law in 1851.[34]

Simon was ecstatic when the Sanitary Act of 1866 was passed. It was the first law of its kind to contain more mandatory compliances than voluntary ones. That fact prompted him to state that it "represented such a stride of advance as virtually to begin a new era." He further commented that "under the Act, the grammar of common sanitary legislation acquired the novel virtue of an imperative mood," and he spoke optimistically concerning the fact "that influences which have hitherto been causing about a quarter of our total mortality are now for the most part brought within control of the law."[35] Simon regarded William Farr's zymotic theory as "the underlying concept that united the new germ theory with the sanitarians' war against filth. Both filth and germ could be seen as contributing causes of disease, filth serving as a medium for the propagation of the disease germ."[36] With Parliament on his side during the 1860s, Simon enjoyed a great deal of success. He established a Medical Department manned by seventeen inspectors who engaged in scientific research on the causes of disease. He persuaded the medical profession to endorse more than fifteen laws designed to improve public health and began the publication of the *Annual Reports* which dealt with existing and future effects of governmental policies. Finally, he was able to personally give the prime minister information on public health. As one historian has noted, that feat was "not achieved again in substance for over two generations."[37]

Eventually, however, tradition and politics led to Simon's ouster from his unique position. In 1876 he angrily vacated his post when his department was combined with the Poor Law Administration under the oversight of the Local Government Board. The Local Government Act of 1871 and the Public Health Act of 1872 had arranged the merger and had created the new agency to supervise it, with a politician named James Stansfeld as its president. He slighted Simon and those who worked for him. "Medical officers were given neither a voice in shaping policy nor encouragement in pursuing research . . . and for years the place of the chief medical officer remained at issue between the profession and the government."[38] As late as 1910, only two years before Lister's death, Sidney and Beatrice Webb argued that the health care provided

[34] Steven J. Novak, "Professionalism and Bureaucracy: English Doctors and the Victorian Public Health Administration," *Journal of Social History* 6 (Summer 1973): 447–49; M. Jeanne Peterson, *The Medical Profession in Mid-Victorian London* (Berkeley: University of California Press, 1978), pp. 34–35; John Simon, *English Sanitary Institutions* (London: Cassell & Company, Limited, 1890), pp. v–vi.

[35] Quoted in Wohl, *Endangered Lives,* p. 156.

[36] Christopher Hamlin, "Providence and Putrefaction: Victorian Sanitarians and the Natural Theology of Health and Disease," *Victorian Studies* 28 (Spring 1985): 386–87.

[37] Roy M. MacLeod, "The Anatomy of State Medicine: Concept and Application," in *Medicine and Science in the 1860s,* ed. F. N. L. Poynter (London: Wellcome Institute for the History of Medicine, 1968), p. 207.

[38] Novak, "Professionalism and Bureaucracy," pp. 451–52; Jeanne L. Brand, "John Simon and the Local Government Board Bureaucrats, 1871–1876," *Bulletin of the History of Medicine* 37 (March–April 1963): 187–88.

by the government was still inadequate because it was restricted by the Poor Law of 1834. In *The State and the Doctor* these Fabian Socialists predicted that the personnel associated with Poor Law infirmaries "would remain a second-class service, for the professionalism of the medical staff suffered from the limitations imposed by confusing the treatment of the sick with the discouraging of pauperism."[39]

Against the backdrop of these events, Lister endeavored to place antisepsis as a doctrine that addressed health concerns in a much more individual, practical way. As one historian has phrased it, "therapeutic nihilism" in the 1850s gave way to "eager expectation of cure," and the British people came to view medical care as a cherished personal right. Lister owed a great deal to those who had fought anticontagionism, to those who had associated specific diseases with specific organisms, and to those whose energies were spent in improving the public's health. In the same year that the Second Reform Act doubled the electorate in Great Britain and redistributed forty-five seats of Parliament in order to provide more representation, Lister started giving his fellow Britons new hope for longevity and a better quality of life.[40]

---

[39] M. A. Crowther, *The Workhouse System, 1834–1929: The History of an English Social Institution* (Athens, Georgia: The University of Georgia Press, 1981), p. 156.
[40] Jeanne L. Brand, *Doctors and the State: The British Medical Profession and Government Action in Public Health, 1870–1912* (Baltimore: The Johns Hopkins University Press, 1965), p. 190.

3. Professional Tradition as a Factor in the Diffusion of Listerism

On March 16, 1867, the first installment of a five-part article entitled "On a New Method of Treating Compound Fracture, Abscess, etc. with Observations on the Conditions of Suppuration" appeared in *The Lancet,* a weekly medical journal published in London. The author of the article was Joseph Lister, a professor of surgery at the University of Glasgow.[1] Four of the parts focused on eleven cases of compound fracture, while the fifth dealt with one of abscess. In the premiere issue Lister said that his new method of treatment, which involved the use of a chemical known as carbolic acid, "afforded results so satisfactory that it does not seem right to withhold it longer from the profession generally."[2]

Carbolic acid is more commonly known as phenol and is a derivative of coal tar. It is a chemical compound consisting of six parts carbon and hydrogen to one part oxygen. The first sample Lister used was in a crude form known as German creosote given to him by Thomas Anderson, a chemistry professor who also taught in Glasgow's university. Lister soon learned, however, that F. Crace-Calvert, an honorary professor of chemistry at Manchester's Royal Institution, owned a factory which refined the substance much more purely and at a fair price. Crace-Calvert had built his business in 1859 and manufactured the acid in the form of white crystals which liquefied at approximately eighty degrees fahrenheit; among its uses had been the preservation of cadavers, but he tried to persuade the medical profession of its other benefits by actively promoting Lister's success with it.[3]

Lister published two additional articles in 1867 entitled "On the Antiseptic Principle in the Practice of Surgery" and "Illustrations of the Antiseptic System of Treatment in Surgery." The author obviously believed he had instituted a system that was based on a scientific principle, that is the germ theory of Louis Pasteur. In the first of these articles, a paper originally presented at the meeting of the British Medical Association in Dublin on August 9, Lister generalized about his major premise by stating, "I arrived, several years ago, at the conclusion that the essential cause of suppuration in wounds is decomposition, brought about by the influence of the atmosphere upon blood or serum retained within them."[4] He was more specific in the second article when he recalled that,

---

[1] Joseph Lister, "On a New Method of Treating Compound Fracture, Abscess, etc. with Observations on the Conditions of Suppuration," *The Lancet* (16 March 1867): 326.

[2] Ibid., (27 July 1867): 95.

[3] Arthur Ernest Sansom, *The Antiseptic System: A Treatise on Carbolic Acid and Its Compounds* (Philadelphia: J. B. Lippincott and Co., 1871), p. 5; Richard B. Fisher, *Joseph Lister, 1827–1912* (New York: Stein and Day, 1977), pp. 121, 134–35; Robert H. Kargon, *Science in Victorian Manchester* (Baltimore: The Johns Hopkins University Press, 1977), pp. 142–43.

[4] Joseph Lister, "On the Antiseptic Principle in the Practice of Surgery," *The Lancet* (21 September 1867): 353; forty years later Lister said that his address in Dublin indicated "how at that very early period the essential principles had been already applied successfully to all departments of surgical practice." Joseph Lister to Hector Clare Cameron, 21 January 1907, Joseph Lister Papers, Library, Royal College of Surgeons of Edinburgh, Edinburgh, GD5, 65.

It is now six years since I first publicly taught in the University of Glasgow that the occurrence of suppuration in a wound under ordinary circumstances, and its continuance on a healthy granulating sore treated with water-dressing, are determined simply by the influence of decomposing organic matter. The subject has since received a large share of my attention, resulting in the system of treatment which I have been engaged for the last three years in elaborating. The benefits which attend this practice are so remarkable that I feel it incumbent upon me to do what I can to diffuse them; and with this view I propose to present to the readers of THE LANCET a series of illustrative cases, prefacing them with a short notice of the principles which it is essential to bear in mind in order to attain success.[5]

Lister's father commented favorably on the readability of his son's writing but was guarded in his assessment of the germ theory. Joseph Jackson Lister, a devout Quaker, said the articles were "very satisfactory (supposing Pasteur's observations to be reliable), & the great success of thy practice based on them tells much in their favour."[6]

In truth, it had been less than three years since Lister initially experimented with carbolic acid as an antiseptic treatment for wounds. Two years to the month before his first article on antisepsis appeared, he had used the acid twice, to perform a wrist excision and to treat a compound fracture of the leg. Though both attempts ended in failure, Lister remained certain of the efficacy of his chosen agent because of a report he had read in 1864 concerning its use in Carlisle, England. It was utilized there to counteract the smell of sewage and to kill infestation detrimental to cattle that were pastured on "land irrigated with the refuse material."[7]

Success finally came to Lister in August, 1865, when he treated another compound fracture "with carbolic acid in its full strength to prevent decomposition." The patient, James Greenlees, was eleven years old, and his left leg had been injured by a cart. Lister first administered the acid to the recesses of the wound by using "a swab" which he held with forceps. Then he placed a piece of lint soaked in the acid over the wound so that it extended onto the uninjured skin. Finally, "a tin cap" was used as a canopy to stop the carbolic from evaporating, and the leg was splinted; Lister recommended "tinfoil strengthened with adhesive plaster" or the "thin sheet-lead used for lining tea-chests" to cover wounds, and he lifted his "cap" every day to pour more acid on the lint. This was done for four days, but because the acid irritated healthy skin surrounding the wound Lister changed to lint saturated with a mixture of water and a small amount of the acid for the next five days. After that he employed an olive-oil solution containing five to ten percent acid for an additional four days and finished with water dressings until healing was complete. Greenlees went home after slightly more than six weeks.[8]

[5] Joseph Lister, "Illustrations of the Antiseptic System of Treatment in Surgery," *The Lancet* (30 November 1867): 668; water dressings had been devised by Robert Liston, who washed wounds with cold water, spaced sutures to provide for drainage, and applied a covering drenched in H_2O. Cuthbert Dukes, *Lord Lister (1827–1912)* (London: Leonard Parsons, 1924), pp. 75–76.

[6] Joseph Jackson Lister to Joseph Lister, 4 December 1867, Western Manuscripts, Wellcome Institute for the History of Medicine, London, MS 6965, 55.

[7] Fisher, *Joseph Lister*, p. 135; Lister, "New Method," (16 March 1867): 327.

[8] Archibald E. Malloch, "Some Memories of Mr. Lister," *Canadian Journal of Medicine and Surgery* 31 (May 1912): 49; Lister, "New Method," (16 March 1867): 327; Lister, "Antiseptic Principle," pp. 353–54.

Few surgeons agreed with Lister's assessment of his success, however, and opponents quickly emerged who were well-prepared to attack his use of carbolic acid as well as Pasteur's germ theory. In an editorial which was to be the first of many on Lister's ideas, *The Lancet* distinguished between the credit due to Pasteur and that due to Lister. It pointed out that the research was the former's work but that the application of the germ theory to compound fractures and abscesses was solely the latter's doing. James G. Wakley, the editor who later became Lister's nemesis, invited supporters and critics to investigate Lister's claims and asked practitioners to confirm them through "further experiment and observation."[9] He also encouraged proponents and adversaries of Lister's approach to vent their feelings in *The Lancet*. Some supported Lister from the beginning, especially in Scotland and on the continent of Europe, but others, particularly in England, tried to discredit him or simply refused to give him a hearing.[10]

One practitioner felt duty-bound to "corroborate" Lister's account with one case of his own and stressed the importance of "all publicity" being given to others which did likewise.[11] Another surgeon bristled at the notion that Lister was the first to use carbolic acid as an agent of healing and blamed wound diseases on "contaminated *hospital air*." The second of these, who was clearly a miasmatist, expressed his belief that the germ theory was "upon debatable ground."[12]

The most virulent attack on Lister's credibility, however, came from James Y. Simpson in the *Edinburgh Daily Review*. Wakley referred to Simpson's article, in which the noted anesthesiologist used the pseudonym "Chirurgicus," and reported that Simpson had credited Jules Lemaire, a physician and pharmacist in Paris, with the adoption of carbolic acid "as a disinfectant and surgical agent" long before Lister's first use of it. According to Wakley, Simpson did pay Lister the backhanded compliment "of having made the agent extensively known" in the United Kingdom.[13] Simpson was the first to use chloroform as an anesthetic and was trying to persuade the British medical profession to practice acupressure, his new technique for stopping arterial bleeding with strategically placed needles.[14] Lister's use of carbolized ligatures to stop bleeding ran counter to Simpson's agenda.[15] Simpson also later advocated the leveling of all large hospitals because of their phenomenally high death rates, at a time when Lister was making them safe havens again.[16] (See Figure 5.)

Simpson essentially accused Lister of plagiarizing ideas developed by Lemaire, and Lemaire did indeed write a paper on coal tar that was published in 1860. In this article Lemaire listed the different constituents of coal tar, including carbolic acid, and reported its effectiveness in disinfecting the atmosphere and improving the healing of

[9] James G. Wakley, "The Surgical Use of Carbolic Acid," *The Lancet* (24 August 1867): 234.

[10] A. J. Youngson, *The Scientific Revolution in Victorian Medicine* (New York: Holmes & Meier, 1979), p. 157.

[11] John Ewens, "Use of Carbolic Acid," *The Lancet* (21 September 1867): 383.

[12] J. R. Wolfe, "On the Use of Carbolic Acid," *The Lancet* (28 September 1867): 410.

[13] James G. Wakley, "Carbolic Acid," *The Lancet* (28 September 1867): 412.

[14] James Y. Simpson, "Notes on Acupressure," *The Lancet* (23 February 1867): 233.

[15] J. Y. Simpson, "Carbolic Acid and Its Compounds in Surgery," *The Lancet* (2 November 1867): 548; The Research Readers of the Scientific Department, comp., *Lister and the Ligature* (New Brunswick, N.J.: Johnson & Johnson, 1925), pp. 7–8.

[16] Michael L. Mason, "Joseph Lister: Hospitalism and the Antiseptic Principle," *Quarterly Bulletin of Northwestern University Medical School* 33 (Spring 1959): 152–55.

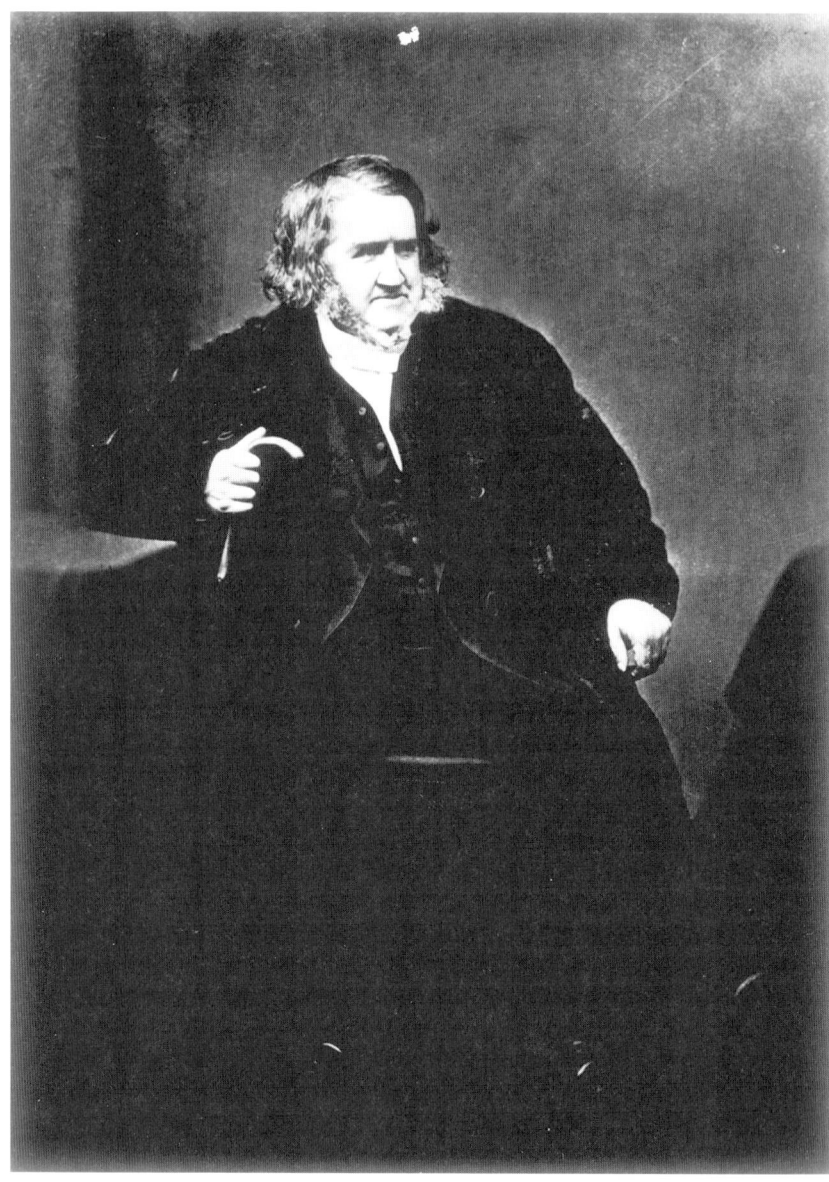

Figure 5. James Y. Simpson

wounds. However, no mention was made of using the substance after surgery, and the use of it during an operation was not done to prevent hospital diseases but to decrease the smell emanating from the discharge of wounds. Lemaire did not believe that the pus itself was diseased, but that it fermented once it was exposed to the air, noting that coal tar stopped the fermentative process and, thus, the production of pus.

Lemaire was a believer in the germ theory and speculated that surgeons who used coal tar to kill what he called "microscopic vegetable organisms which exist in abundance in the atmosphere" might discover something new that would benefit humanity. His strongest support for the germ theory came in a book he authored on carbolic acid in 1863. There, Lemaire recommended the chemical for every conceivable ailment and simply assumed that germs had been destroyed in those patients who recovered. No method or guiding principle was proposed for the use of carbolic acid, and even though "Lemaire realized what the causes of putrefaction were . . . he made no attempt to exclude them, nor indeed did he make any systematic attempts to eradicate them after they had entered."[17]

In the first issue of *The Lancet* for October, 1867, Lister responded to Simpson's reference to Lemaire. He denied ever having heard of the Parisian practitioner or of his work, and argued that even in France Lemaire had not caused enough of a stir to prompt the medical profession to react and had not had any tangible impact on the healing art. After minimizing Lemaire's significance, Lister squarely positioned himself for battle with his critics by confidently announcing,

> For my own part, I may say that, of all the gentlemen from Great Britain and both continents who have recently visited Glasgow, not one has ever expressed the slightest doubt that the system in question was entirely new; the novelty, I may remark, being, not the surgical use of carbolic acid (which I never claimed), but the methods of its employment with the view of protecting the reparatory processes from disturbance by external agency.[18]

Lister went on to enumerate the ways his method had been disparaged: first, his choice of antiseptics had been categorized as "useless," and second, his application of it had not been viewed as "original." These criticisms he labeled "unworthy cavils."[19] One week later some encouraging news from King's College Hospital of London was reported in *The Lancet*. It said that carbolic acid had been widely used in that institution by assistant surgeons to stop pus from forming in patient's wounds and had been "followed by very successful results."[20] Not only must this have lifted Lister's spirits, but also it indicated that some in England were at least aware of his work.

Perhaps inspired by the King's College results, Lister continued to defend himself against Simpson's attacks. He had found a copy of Lemaire's book on the use of carbolic acid and had determined that it was testimony to the "insignificance of the results" attained by its author. Lister reiterated that he had at no time laid claim to being the first physician to use the substance in the operating theater. He said he chose carbolic acid because of its strength, but confidently noted that similar findings could have been rendered with any number of disinfectants which had "analogous properties," if they had been applied following his recommended methods. He warned surgeons to "not expect carbolic acid to act like a charm."

[17] W. Watson Cheyne, *Antiseptic Surgery: Its Principles, Practice, History and Results* (London: Smith, Elder, & Co., 1882), pp. 352–55.

[18] Joseph Lister, "On the Use of Carbolic Acid," *The Lancet* (5 October 1867): 444; actually, Lemaire's book was issued in a second edition only two years after it was originally published, and contrary to Lister's appraisal there was "interest excited in France." Cheyne, *Antiseptic Surgery,* p. 355.

[19] Lister, "Carbolic Acid," p. 444.

[20] James G. Wakley, "King's College Hospital," *The Lancet* (12 October 1867): 455.

Lister amplified his remarks by including a letter from a medical student who lived in Carlisle, the town which had treated its sewage with carbolic acid. The student, Philip Hair, related that he had spent the previous winter in Paris and that he had seen nothing comparable to Lister's method practiced in the French capital. He did observe the use of phenic acid, an extremely diluted form of the agent used by Lister, but only for the purpose of washing wounds. Additionally, Hair had offered the testimony of eight other students to substantiate his account.[21] The fact that Lister used the testimonial of an obscure medical student to support his arguments illustrates how alone he was in the world of surgery.

Lister's defense of his system and his willingness to respond to famous critics apparently further angered James Y. Simpson, who was professor of medicine and midwifery at the University of Edinburgh. Simpson, in an effort to demolish Lister, prepared an article on carbolic acid under his own name instead of under the pseudonym "Chirurgicus." In it he again alluded to Lemaire as well as others in France and the German states who had worked with carbolic acid several years before Lister, but he showed how little attention he had paid to Lister's words when he cited the report of a correspondent for *The Lancet* who had been investigating surgical practices in Paris. That correspondent, Sampson Gamgee, did report seeing surgeons use a solution of carbolic acid, but one that was far more diluted than what Lister had recommended; one part of the acid was combined with one-hundred parts water, whereas Lister now suggested a ratio of one to forty.

Simpson's true motive emerged in the last two paragraphs of his article where he compared the use of acupressure to that of ligatures treated with carbolic acid to stop arterial bleeding. He singled out William Pirrie, of the University of Aberdeen Hospital, as an example of one who employed acupressure to stop the formation of pus in two-thirds of his cases involving the removal of tumors from breasts. Furthermore, after chastising Lister for referring to his antiseptic results as "magnificent," Simpson bragged that there had been no pyemia at the hospital since the practice of acupressure began and compared its death rate from amputation to those of both Glasgow and Edinburgh.[22]

To Simpson's embarrassment, this attack on Lister was followed one week later by an article written by none other than Professor Pirrie. Pirrie extolled the virtues of carbolic acid for the treatment of burns and volunteered the fact that it had proven effective in other ailments. He further predicted, "If in other cases of the same degrees of burn carbolic acid should be equally useful, it would be a great blessing in the treatment of these dangerous and painful injuries."[23] As it turned out, Lister had not waited for Pirrie's response to Simpson's renewed attack, but had quickly prepared his own reply. In it he acknowledged Simpson's "allegations," and asked the readers of *The Lancet* "to judge for themselves how far the present attack admits of justification," promising to publish additional articles on his antiseptic technique.[24]

Although Simpson's attacks on Lister were partly motivated by his desire to pro-

[21] Lister, "Carbolic Acid," (19 October 1867): 502.
[22] Simpson, "Carbolic Acid," p. 548–49.
[23] William Pirrie, "On the Use of Carbolic Acid in Burns," *The Lancet* (9 November 1867): 575.
[24] Lister, "Carbolic Acid," (9 November 1867): 595.

mote his acupressure system, he soon attracted supporters such as Frederick W. Ricketts, a young physician from Liverpool. Ricketts, while hesitant to "enter the list with learned professors and magnates," nevertheless sided with Simpson and others who viewed the use of carbolic acid as descended from the traditional practice of putting any number of ointments on the raw surfaces of wounds in a very unscientific manner. He found acupressure "simple, effectual, and elegant," but viewed Lister's method as "obsolete and inelegant." He ended his review of the subject by expressing his wish that the issue would "not be allowed to rest till decisive and authoritative statements be given."[25]

In mid-December, 1867, two powerful letters were printed in *The Lancet* which helped put the ongoing argument in perspective. The first was from Arthur Hensman, a young surgeon like Ricketts, who reminded the British medical profession that the use of carbolic acid had become less and less frequent prior to Lister's success with it. Thus, he credited Lister with establishing the truth which others had overlooked. As far as contrary opinions were concerned, he passionately spoke of the fact that he would feel "almost criminal" if he let them dissuade him from a successful practice.[26] The second boldly declared that none of the efforts to "overthrow" Lister had succeeded, and that both he and Simpson had devised original techniques for healing suppurative wounds. The originality was not in the agents used, whether carbolic acid or needles, but in the way they were employed.[27]

With the new year came new attacks and a new strategy conceived to destroy the principle on which the antiseptic system was founded. On January 17, 1868, John Hughes Bennett delivered a speech to the Royal College of Surgeons in Edinburgh entitled "The Atmospheric Germ Theory." Bennett, Professor of the Institutes of Medicine and Senior Professor of Clinical Medicine at the University of Edinburgh, never mentioned Lister in his address. He did, however, challenge Pasteur's experiments which had led to the germ theory. In Bennett's words,

> The theory of atmospheric germs . . . has been ably sustained by M. Pasteur, who, by new experiments, has revived the doctrine that fermentation and putrefaction are not chemical processes . . . but physiological phenomena dependent on living germs derived from the atmosphere. These experiments gained for him, in 1859, the Grand Prize for Physiology annually awarded by the French Academy of Sciences. They have all, however, been since repeated by Pouchet and others, and their accuracy as well as the correctness of his conclusions are by them utterly denied.[28]

More than once Bennett alluded to the fact that Pasteur was a chemist and in one sentence indicted all French chemists in a very condescending manner. He rejected Pasteur's methodology out of hand because it did not meet the accepted standards of the medical profession, especially in terms of temperatures applied to infusions, liquid

[25] Frederick W. Ricketts, "On the Use of Carbolic Acid," *The Lancet* (16 November 1867): 614.
[26] Arthur Hensman, "On the Use of Carbolic Acid," *The Lancet* (14 December 1867): 757.
[27] John Dewar, "On the Use of Carbolic Acid," *The Lancet* (14 December 1867): 757.
[28] John Hughes Bennett, "The Atmospheric Germ Theory," *Edinburgh Medical Journal* 13 (March 1868): 812.

suspensions of decaying organic matter used as culture media. Instead, he insisted that molecules visible on top of the cultures, "out of which animalcules and fungi are produced, are not derived from the air. Neither can they be supposed to preexist in the fluid, as then they would be readily seen, which they never are at the commencement." To resolve the obvious difference between his view and that of Pasteur, Bennett proposed what he called "the process of molecular coalescence."[29]

In his final paragraph Bennett succinctly explained his theory which he called "truth," supported by no less than the ancient Greeks and the Holy Scriptures:

> The truth seems to be, that new life springs from the molecular death of pre-existing tissues and organisms. The vibratile and germinal molecules concerned in the process are not new productions, but old ones, and these, submitted to conditions which it is the office of the physiologist to investigate, undergo a rejuvenescence, and enter into and constitute the living substance of the new being. This theory, I venture to think, is not only consistent with all known facts, but unites in one grand conclusion the physiological science of the present day, the intellectual speculations of ancient Greece, and the direct teachings of our sacred records.[30]

To argue with Bennett was to take issue with Democritus and the apostle Paul. However, Lister was told by his own father that it was not important "to defend the Germ Theory, which might be left to take care of itself, but to describe distinctly the *Treatment* adopted by thee (which that theory *suggested*)." He also advised his son "to show by *Cases* the remarkable results of thy treatment with its progressive improvements, in *contrast to* those results which follow the *usual* course of practice."[31]

Regardless of the germ theory's veracity, Bennett's convoluted arguments were more than many practitioners could tolerate. A physician from New Zealand said it best when he reminded his fellows that Lister's technique should be put in "the hands of every practitioner . . . who has the advancement of 'conservative surgery' and the interests of his patients at heart." He described Lister, under whom he had studied for two years, as a "philosophic surgeon" and, being bolder than his teacher, claimed that on first and second degree burns carbolic acid did work "almost like a charm."[32] His reference to "conservative surgery" was taken from Hensman, who said it would essentially be a crime not to adopt Lister's system, and his description of Lister was directed at Simpson who had used the same two-word label in what was apparently considered a derogatory manner.

Another of Lister's former students, who wrote from Java, included the antiseptic system in what he called "startling novelties" that had brought about "changes of and additions to our former theories and practice." He even posed a question for the contemplation of his "professional brethren," which opened the door for continued em-

---

[29] Ibid., pp. 822, 831.
[30] Ibid., pp. 833–34.
[31] Joseph Jackson Lister to Joseph Lister, 20 March 1868, Western Manuscripts, Wellcome Institute for the History of Medicine, London, MS 6965, 59.
[32] J. Rutherford Ryley, "Carbolic Acid in the Treatment of Compound Fractures and Abscesses," *The Lancet* (9 May 1868): 586–87.

phasis on the agent to the exclusion of the principle behind its use: "May the carbolic acid treatment not yet prove to be the best agent for the treatment of even extensive joint disease?"[33]

If more proof of the success associated with the use of carbolic acid as a medical cleansing agent was needed, it was furnished in an overwhelmingly effective way by Pearson R. Cresswell, chief surgeon of the Dowlais Iron Works in Merthyr Tydfil. The business in South Wales employed more than eighty-five hundred workers, and Cresswell treated all types of injuries with the substance, "in every instance with marked success." He characterized the impact of carbolic acid on surgery as "quite a revolution."[34] This prompted the editor of *The Lancet* to wonder aloud why Lister's method had not enjoyed favorable results in London. He asked, "Are the conditions of suppuration different here from those in Glasgow or Dowlais? Or is it that the antiseptic treatment is not tried with that care without which Mr. Lister has always pointed out it does not succeed?"[35] Six weeks after asking these questions, he stated that Lister was "generally imitated" in the United Kingdom and expressed the hope that his system would "abide the best of trials—viz., the trial of time."[36] That news may have led to a clever about-face by Lister's father, who now counseled his son that his next article should "serve as a summary & inform the profession that the operations given are not *exceptional* but *examples,* (striking ones) of a *usual* course of success."[37]

Following Wakley's inquiries, reports from various London physicians began occupying the pages of *The Lancet* for several months. Some of them were long overdue admissions of positive accomplishments with Lister's technique, while others clearly manifested carelessness and ignorance in implementing it. C. F. Maunder, a surgeon employed at the London Hospital, wrote that he had used the antiseptic method with ligatures, concluding with his belief that "the antiseptic ligature of arteries will greatly diminish the risk of secondary haemorrhage."[38] In an article highlighting St. George's Hospital, Wakley stated that Lister's plan had been tried "pretty extensively" in London and that he had asked its hospitals to report on their experience with it. However, since the information they had supplied was insufficient to commend or impugn the antiseptic technique, he cautiously added, "It is probably as yet too soon for a very decided opinion to be pronounced upon its merits."[39]

It was not long, though, before reports from the hospitals began to arrive. Middlesex Hospital recorded some success with the use of carbolic acid and noted that, "As an ordinary lotion, it is the most frequently prescribed, probably, of any of the lotions in common use for dressing wounds and sores, healthy or unhealthy." It must be remembered, concluded the Middlesex surgeons that like every disinfectant, "considerable misconception appears to exist with reference to the powers of carbolic

---

[33] J. R. Wylie, "Prof. Lister's Treatment of Wounds and Ulcers by Carbolic Acid," *The Lancet* (4 July 1868): 5–6.

[34] Pearson R. Cresswell, "Case of Gunshot Wound of the Left Hip Treated on the Antiseptic Principle; Recovery.," *The Lancet* (29 August 1868): 277.

[35] James G. Wakley, "Compound Comminuted Fracture of Femur without a Trace of Suppuration," *The Lancet* (5 September 1868): 324.

[36] James G. Wakley, "Antiseptic Surgery," *The Lancet* (17 October 1868): 520.

[37] Joseph Jackson Lister to Joseph Lister, 10 November 1868, Western Manuscripts, Wellcome Institute for the History of Medicine, London, MS 6965, 61.

[38] C. F. Maunder, "On the Antiseptic Ligature of Arteries," *The Lancet* (7 November 1868): 596.

[39] James G. Wakley, "St. George's Hospital," *The Lancet* (14 November 1868): 634.

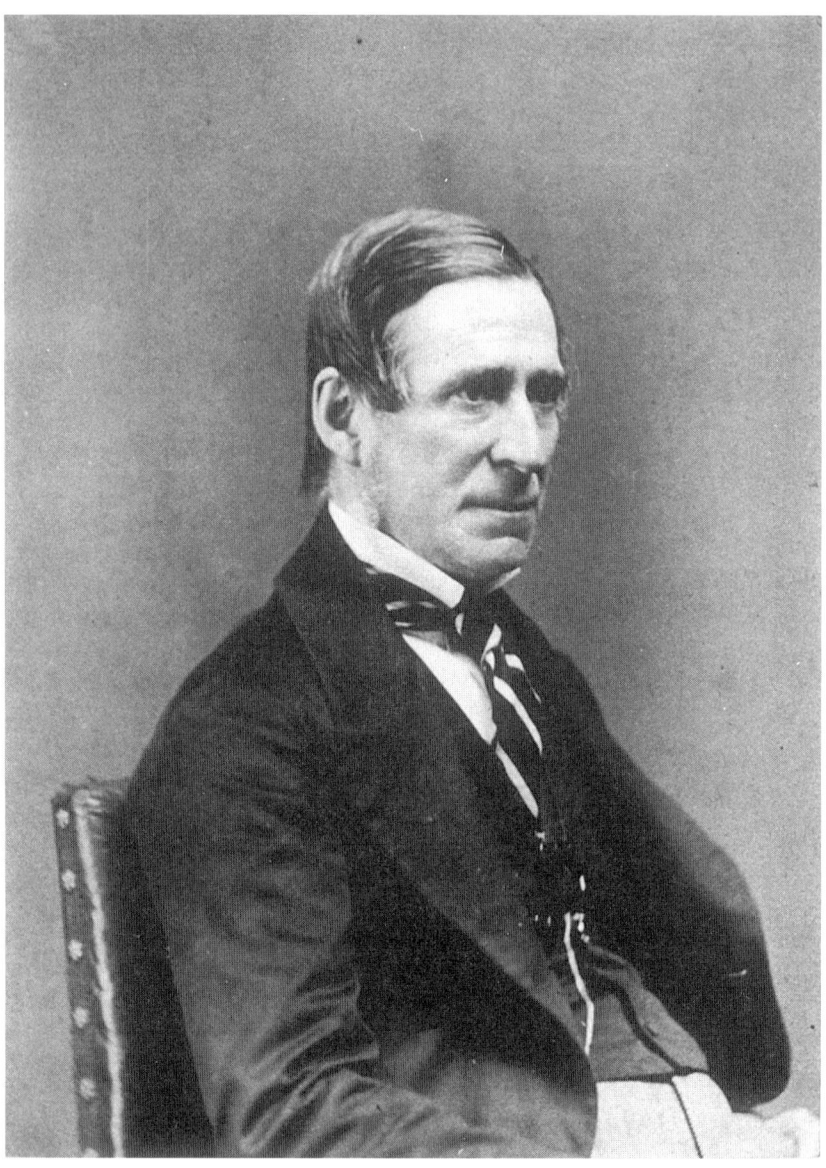
Figure 6. James Paget

acid."[40] The inconsistency experienced in London's smaller hospitals was also shared by two of the capital's leading institutions, St. Bartholomew's Hospital and Guy's Hospital.

James Paget, one of the most highly regarded surgeons in London, who practiced at St. Bartholomew's until 1878, had not completely made up his mind about Lister's method but admitted that he had found carbolic acid "useless." (See Figure 6.) He

---

[40] James G. Wakley, "Middlesex Hospital," *The Lancet* (28 November 1868): 695.

was willing to concede, though, that he might be applying it wrong.[41] Another surgeon at St. Bartholomew's Hospital rejected Lister's approach because he found it to be "meddlesome." He and a colleague at Guy's Hospital preferred to continue treating wounds according to "the usual plan," which meant employing an open method whereby the edges of wounds were left unapproximated to heal, or not to heal, on their own.[42] Why this strategy enjoyed the relative success it did in the nineteenth century has never been definitively answered. "Free drainage of wound secretions, the drying influence of exposure to air, and a wound temperature approximating that of the room are likely determinants responsible for the decreased replication of microorganisms under these conditions."[43]

Thomas Bryant, the chief surgeon at Guy's Hospital, had repeatedly tried Lister's treatment in order to heal wounds and, for the most part, had positive outcomes which he was "disposed to attribute . . . in a great measure to the use of the carbolic acid." Yet, success was not certain. According to an article by Thomas Stevenson, also of Guy's Hospital, carbolic acid was responsible for the death of one of Bryant's patients. A female amputee had urinated approximately two ounces of a black-colored fluid just prior to her death. Stevenson observed that the woman's stump had been dressed with carbolic acid and that "it is a singular circumstance that in nearly all cases in which true black urine has been passed, either wood—or coal-tar creosote—both of which contain carbolic acid or closely allied bodies—has been administered either externally or internally."[44]

John Wood, another London surgeon, experimented widely with diverse types of carbolic acid combinations at King's College Hospital. He alternately mixed it with water, oil, and in putty. His experience with the last of these three proved effective in most instances, but ineffective in a significant minority of cases. As a possible explanation for his varied results, Wood noted that the decreased benefits of the acid corresponded to a worsening of the sanitation of the institution. In the fall of the year,

> the hospital air became vitiated; and notwithstanding the free use of carbolic acid in the waterclosets and wards, and in the water used for all purposes of ablution and disinfection, many of the cases treated with carbolic acid in exactly the same careful way resulted in free suppuration.[45]

Lister had already introduced the use of "a firm putty" in the fall of the previous year, only months after authoring his first article on the antiseptic method. He made it by mixing carbonate of lime with a one to four solution of carbolic acid and boiled linseed oil. It kept enough of the acid around the wound to stop decay from spreading

[41] Stephen Paget, ed., *Memoirs and Letters of Sir James Paget* (London: Longmans, Green and Co., 1901) p. 357; James G. Wakley, "The Use of Carbolic Acid," *The Lancet* (5 December 1868): 728.

[42] Irving I. Edgar, "Modern Surgery and Lord Lister," *Journal of the History of Medicine and Allied Sciences* 16 (April 1961): 148; Wakley, "The Use of Carbolic Acid," p. 728.

[43] Owen H. Wangensteen, Jacqueline Smith, and Sarah D. Wangensteen, "Some Highlights in the History of Amputation Reflecting Lessons in Wound Healing," *Bulletin of the History of Medicine* 41 (March–April 1967): 117.

[44] Thomas Stevenson, "Note on a Case of Melanuria," *Guy's Hospital Reports,* Third Series, 13 (1868): 407–08; Wakley, "The Use of Carbolic Acid," p. 728.

[45] Wakley, "King's College," (12 December 1868): 762.

internally but not so much that the adjacent healthy surface sloughed; undiluted carbolic acid had limited the amount of skin that could be covered.[46]

Wood based his endeavors on the work of both Lister and James Syme because he not only took steps to exclude dangerous particles from the air, but also applied full-strength carbolic acid in certain cases to facilitate the formation of scabs. For scabbing, its "efficacy, manageability, cleanliness, and rapidity of results" were "infinitely superior to any other escharotic that has been tried."[47] Occasionally, "a sort of thick . . . putty, made of the acid mixed with oil" was also tested at Charing-Cross Hospital. The surgeon who implemented it there, however, was unwilling to invest the time necessary to make the plaster on a routine basis, not recognizing that it would later save him labor and possibly his patient's life.[48]

The last of the London hospitals to present evidence relative to the employment of the antiseptic method was University College Hospital, where Lister had earned his medical degree in 1852. Again, the findings were mixed. Great success had been achieved in certain cases and complete failure was experienced in others. The general consensus was that, caught early enough, there were fewer complications and less suppuration in wounds treated with carbolic acid, though the time necessary for healing was not appreciably shortened. London surgeons seemed to agree, however, that once the presence of pus was "established" and "confirmed" the antiseptic technique was "productive of nothing but harm."[49]

Although surgeons at University College had not had complete success in using carbolic acid to prevent suppuration, they did report one spectacular success. The most dreaded complications from surgery in a hospital setting were pyemia, a form of blood poisoning caused by bacteria, and erysipelas, an infectious disease caused by a streptococcus. According to the University College Hospital report,

> It so happened that during the earlier months of last year, pyaemia was exceedingly rife in this hospital. Patient after patient perished by it; and indeed recovery after amputation of a limb was almost becoming an exceptional rarity. This endemic of pyaemia continued up to the date at which carbolic-acid dressings began to be used. Not one of those treated antiseptically died of pyaemia, or indeed ever had a pyaemic symptom.
> Phlegmonous erysipelas has not once occurred here in connection with antiseptic dressings in the wards.[50]

Events in London, of course, were carefully watched by physicians outside the capital. Having read the numerous accounts from there, John Rose, a surgeon at Kidderminster Infirmary in western England, was inspired to report his own experience

---

[46] Lister, "Antiseptic Principle," p. 354.
[47] Wakley, "King's College," (12 December 1868): 763; the earliest biography of Syme points out that he was a surgeon in the University of Edinburgh's Hospital, the leading opponent of acupressure, a foe of John Hughes Bennett, and Lister's father-in-law. Robert Paterson, *Memorials of the Life of James Syme* (Edinburgh: Edmonston and Douglas, 1874), pp. 261–63, 264–66.
[48] James G. Wakley, "Charing-Cross Hospital," *The Lancet* (9 January 1869): 47.
[49] James G. Wakley, "University College Hospital," *The Lancet* (16 January 1869): 86–87.
[50] Ibid., p. 86.

with carbolic acid. He quickly praised it "as one of the most useful of modern thera-peutic agents in surgical practice" and stressed that "a vast amount of misery, discom-fort, and mutilation" had been alleviated. Much of his practice was with limbs severed in industrial mishaps, and the use of carbolic acid allowed him to avoid many ampu-tations. "Since its introduction," he said, "our operations have been less numerous, although accidents from machinery and other causes have been on the increase, and of almost daily occurrence."[51]

Irish surgeons were also aware of what was happening in London, and one, in particular, stepped to the forefront with astute, common sense observations for his brotherhood. William MacCormac, who practiced at Belfast General Hospital, put the controversy over Lister's system of treatment in perspective by saying that, "were it only partially to accomplish all that it assumes to accomplish, [it] would rank amongst the greatest surgical achievements of our day."[52] After listing eight cases in which he had successfully implemented the system, he concluded with a succinct analysis of the germ theory and Lister's application of it to surgery:

> The theory that Professor Lister offers to account for all this is one of great sim-plicity, and one which so far explains the facts observed, and until one more satisfactory be offered, we are perhaps bound to accept it. However, be it true or false, by acting strictly in accordance with its requirements, the surgeon will, I believe, procure results which he could not otherwise have anticipated.[53]

Once the parade of articles pertaining to London hospitals stopped, Lister began to write for *The Lancet* again himself. He reemerged on its pages in response to a published lecture by the eminent James Paget, who had now apparently decided to reject most aspects of the antiseptic technique. Paget still accepted blame for his fail-ures with carbolic acid but saw great potential for harm in using it, attributing detri-mental effects to "leaving it too long when the wound should have been left open to discharge itself." Usually, Lister refuted claims of this sort by accusing their authors of carelessness. Paget anticipated this argument by maintaining that he had followed List-er's plan, "if not with all the skill that Professor Lister would employ it, yet with more than is ever likely to be generally used in the treatment of fractures; and yet it certainly did no good."[54]

Lister, who had sworn off defending himself from James Simpson because Simp-son's responses had degenerated into personal attacks, could not ignore this James, who had previously been balanced in his appraisal of the antiseptic system and whose opinion was respected more than that of any other surgeon in London. In a measured reply, Lister stated "that the practice followed in this instance had very little in com-mon with anything that I have advised." Paget had used collodion, soluble guncotton dissolved in a mixture of ether and alcohol, to cover the wound before applying a

---

[51] John Rose, "On the Use of Carbolic Acid in Compound Fractures, Wounds, Burns, and Gunshot Wounds," *The Lancet* (16 January 1869): 89.

[52] William MacCormac, "On the Antiseptic Treatment of Wounds," *The Dublin Journal of Medical Science* 47 (February 1869): 52.

[53] Ibid., pp. 61–62.

[54] James Paget, "Clinical Lecture on the Treatment of Fractures of the Leg," *The Lancet* (6 March 1869): 317.

carbolic-acid putty twelve hours later. The use of collodion to seal wounds was known as the occlusion method, which Lister had rejected because it did not permit drainage. In spite of the difference in what Paget did and what strict adherence to the antiseptic technique required, Lister's final paragraph explained the reason for his caution in confronting Paget. "Had this lecture," he said,

> proceeded from anyone less deservedly eminent than Mr. Paget, I should not have felt called upon to notice it. But as anything from such an authority is calculated to have great influence with the profession, I have felt reluctantly compelled to allude to the matter thus publicly.[55]

Undeterred, Lister continued to refine his technique. He used a drainage tube made from India rubber on a patient whose forearm had been amputated, for example.[56] Such tubes had first been employed ten years before by a French surgeon named Edouard Chassaignac, but Lister was apparently unaware of his work. Lister's biographers have been equally unfamiliar with their subject's earliest use of this medical advance. They attribute his initial experience with drainage tubes to the time when he operated on Queen Victoria for an abscess, two-and-a-half years later. Presumably, they do this because Lister's own recollection of events may have been inaccurate.[57] Nearly four decades after utilizing a rubber tube on the unnamed amputee, Lister reminisced that he had used lint wicks for drainage until 1871, when he opened a six-inch long abscess on his most famous patient. Her name defined an entire age. Possibly, he suffered from a lapse of memory, but he could have been specifically pointing out when he first used rubber drains in abscesses as opposed to other surgeries. It only stands to reason that he would not have conducted an untried experiment on the monarch.[58]

While his use of rubber tubes for drainage in 1869 went unheralded by him and his disciples, Lister did submit articles to *The Lancet* that year describing a new way to approach an ancient practice that had fallen into disuse. He reintroduced sutures made from naturally-absorbed catgut, instead of relying on traditional ligatures made from unspun silk. When he administered them antiseptically, they caused the healing of arteries to occur more rapidly. Their absorption did not have to be feared when their use was based on Lister's principle; after they disappeared there would be nothing left to cause irritation, and the carbolic acid in which they were steeped would continue to benefit the patient. Catgut is made from the small intestines of sheep, is inexpensive compared to other ligatures, and is very strong. Summarizing its boon to

---

[55] Joseph Lister, "The Antiseptic Treatment of Compound Fracture," *The Lancet* (13 March 1869): 380; guncotton is made by digesting clean cotton in a mixture of one part nitric acid and three parts sulfuric acid. Edgar, "Modern Surgery," p. 148.

[56] Joseph Jackson Lister to Joseph Lister, 27 January 1869, Western Manuscripts, Wellcome Institute for the History of Medicine, London, MS 6965, 63.

[57] Rickman John Godlee, *Lord Lister*, 3d ed. (Oxford: The Clarendon Press, 1924), pp. 303–304; Hector Charles Cameron, *Joseph Lister: The Friend of Man* (London: William Heinemann, 1949), pp. 7–9; Fisher, *Joseph Lister*, pp. 193–94; F. F. Cartwright, "Antiseptic Surgery," in *Medicine and Science in the 1860s*, ed. F. N. L. Poynter (London: Wellcome Institute for the History of Medicine, 1968), pp. 80, 96–97.

[58] Lord Lister, "Remarks on Some Points in the History of Antiseptic Surgery," *The Lancet* (27 June 1908): 1815; Christopher Hibbert, ed., *Queen Victoria in her Letters and Journals* (New York: Viking, 1984), pp. 225–26.

surgery, Lister said "that by applying a ligature of animal tissue antiseptically upon an artery, whether tightly or gently, we virtually surround it with a ring of living tissue, and strengthen the vessel where we obstruct it." It is still the ligature chosen by "a goodly percentage of surgeons" in every operating room for some tissues, and Lister's adaptation of it has been extolled as "one of the most practical innovations ever made in technical surgery."[59]

Four days after Lister's article on ligatures appeared in *The Lancet,* Joseph Bell, assistant surgeon at the Royal Infirmary of Edinburgh, read a paper entitled "Cases Illustrative of the Antiseptic Use of Carbolic Acid" to the Medico-Chirurgical Society of that city. In it he described three cases of abscess, one of compound fracture, one of compound dislocation of the elbow joint, two of injury to large joints, and four of amputation, all of which had been successfully treated. He also detailed one of James Syme's amputations, which was far more astounding than any of his in its recovery.[60] In his last paragraph, Bell seemed to agree with William MacCormac, the surgeon from Belfast who had said that the antiseptic system was one of the most significant accomplishments in the nineteenth century, regardless of whether all of its intended goals were ever realized. "Even if on theoretical grounds," Bell cogently surmised,

> surgeons may deny the possibility of preventing suppuration, and ignore our facts, still, if it be granted that by this method we can diminish the amount and destroy the foetor of pus, we have done much to improve the sanitary condition, and diminish the fatality, of our great hospitals.[61]

By 1869 Lister had become controversial enough to provide a convenient target for all those who wished to defend tradition and preconceived ideas, and each of his challenges only elicited renewed animosity by those who thought he was a pretentious charlatan. Even his recommendation for the use of catgut did not escape attack. James Spence, another Edinburgh surgeon, tried carbolized catgut but determined that it was "liable to become altered, softened, and disintegrated by the heat and moisture of the living tissues around it, and thus allow the deligated vessel to become again permeable." He did acknowledge that silk or linen thread prepared with carbolic acid might "be perfectly safe," but his experience was with "ordinary" ligatures which had never come off of an artery like carbolized catgut had.[62]

E. R. Bickersteth, a surgeon at the Liverpool Royal Infirmary, disagreed and took "pleasure" in reporting cases in which he had effectively utilized "the antiseptic catgut ligature." He called the attention of his readers to the fact that, chronologically, his patients were the first to be treated with it.[63] He also related that James Paget had seen

---

[59] Joseph Lister, "Observations on Ligature of Arteries on the Antiseptic System," *The Lancet* (3 April 1869): 451, 455; T. Gibson, "Evolution of catgut ligatures: the endeavours and success of Joseph Lister and William Macewen," *The British Journal of Surgery* 77 (July 1990): 824–25; Sherwin B. Nuland, *Doctors: The Biography of Medicine* (New York: Alfred A. Knopf, 1988), pp. 382–83.

[60] Joseph Bell, "Cases Illustrative of the Antiseptic Use of Carbolic Acid," *Edinburgh Medical Journal* 14 (May 1869): 982–88.

[61] Ibid., p. 988.

[62] James Spence, "On the Use of Carbolized Catgut Ligatures," *The Lancet* (5 June 1869): 772–73.

[63] E. R. Bickersteth, "Remarks on the Antiseptic Treatment of Wounds," *The Lancet* (29 May 1869): 743.

them and "expressed himself as much gratified in witnessing what he termed 'these brilliant results' from the antiseptic ligature and dressings." Personally, Bickersteth expressed his conviction that Lister's method was "an immense step towards the perfection of our art."[64]

Citing Bickersteth's cases in a letter to the managers of the Edinburgh Royal Infirmary, James Syme defended Lister's ligatures and his own house-surgeon, Edward Lawrie, who had been fired for correspondence he submitted to *The Lancet* which refuted James Spence's claims regarding the dangers of using catgut. Lister's father-in-law referred to the administration of the infirmary as a "reign of terror." Ostensibly, Lawrie was dismissed for endeavoring to correct a mistake which had led to Spence's failure with carbolized catgut. Spence had acquired the ligature he used from Lawrie, who thought it met accepted standards, but later realized it was inadequately prepared.[65] Lawrie wrote the managers in his own defense and told them that he had informed Spence of the substandard nature of the ligature which he had furnished "before Mr. Spence wrote his article on the Ligature of the Carotid Artery."[66] The following day, S. G. Littlejohn, resident physician in the clinical wards of the infirmary, resigned because he felt "so strongly the gross injustice which has been done Mr. Lawrie."[67]

Bickersteth also took Spence to task, accusing him of making declarations relevant to carbolized catgut ligature "calculated seriously to prejudice the minds of all operating surgeons against its use, by causing distrust in its safety."[68] Spence did not sit quietly by and ignore the onslaught of articles in opposition to him, but his replies were not adequate to quell criticism. Of Lawrie's letter to *The Lancet,* Spence said that it "contains assertions and insinuations inconsistent with fact."[69] When asked by Lawrie to write him a personal letter outlining these, Spence refused.[70] In addition, the only reference Spence made to Bickersteth's article was that it contained "misstatements."[71]

There were, undoubtedly, inaccuracies on the part of both sides in the prolonged debate over the antiseptic principle. The most publicly damaging of these to Lister's cause came from an English surgeon, Thomas Nunneley. He practiced in the General Infirmary in Leeds and delivered the address on surgery at the annual meeting of the British Medical Association, which was held there on July 27–30, 1869.[72] Nunneley was respected for his study of erysipelas and was "a very intelligent, research-minded surgeon," but he took great pride in stating that he had not permitted a single patient

---

[64] Ibid., (12 June 1869): 811–12; in 1875 Paget said that his greatest pleasure had come from surgical advances "which have not only diminished the mortality after operations, but have diminished the fever and all the other troubles apt to follow them," and while not presuming to rank those improvements in importance, he nonetheless mentioned antisepsis first in a list that included such things as acupressure, carbolized catgut ligatures, healthier hospitals, and cleanliness. James Paget, *Clinical Lectures and Essays,* ed. Howard Marsh (New York: D. Appleton & Company, 1875), pp. 51, 76.

[65] James Syme, "The Managers of the Royal Infirmary and Mr. Lawrie," *The Lancet* (26 June 1869): 888.

[66] Edward Lawrie, "The Managers of the Royal Infirmary and Mr. Lawrie," *The Lancet* (3 July 1869): 29.

[67] S. G. Littlejohn, "The Managers of the Royal Infirmary and Mr. Lawrie," *The Lancet* (3 July 1869): 29.

[68] E. R. Bickersteth, "Carbolized Catgut Ligature," *The Lancet* (24 July 1869): 142.

[69] James Spence, "The Managers of the Royal Infirmary and Mr. Lawrie," *The Lancet* (26 June 1869): 888.

[70] Ibid., (3 July 1869): 29–30.

[71] James Spence, "Carbolized Catgut Ligature," *The Lancet* (31 July 1869): 186.

[72] James G. Wakley, "Report of the Thirty-Seventh Annual Meeting of the British Medical Association," *The Lancet* (7 August 1869): 211.

of his to be treated with carbolic acid. He admitted that his fellow physicians had used the substance, but he confidently proclaimed that their results had been no better than his, and that putting carbolic acid on wounds had become the exception to the rule in Leeds. To support his aversion to antiseptics, he referred to the previous comments of James Y. Simpson and John Hughes Bennett, both of whom were in attendance at the meeting, and emphatically announced that they had "never dreamed of applying antiseptic treatment for the destruction of septic germs."[73]

The dreamers, according to Nunneley, were those who looked to the antiseptic treatment for a cure. He labeled Lister's method as "fashionable" and "in vogue," based on "unsupported fancies, which have little other existence than what is found in the imagination of those who believe in them." Furthermore, he struck at the premise on which Lister's system was based and attempted to drive home his central theme in a very impassioned manner. He pleaded,

> This speculation of organic germs is, I fear, far more than an innocent fallacy; it is a positive injury, for, teaching, as it does, that those desperate consequences which so often follow wounds result from one cause alone, and are to be prevented by attending to it alone, and that in a very simple manner, it leads to the ignoring of those many and often complicated causes, which I have indicated as influencing, for good or evil, the progress of a wounded person, attention to which has hitherto been considered to be one of the most essential parts of a surgeon's duty, and, as achieved or not, in a great degree to distinguish the able and skilful practitioner from the inexperience [*sic*] and unskilful [*sic*] man.[74]

The editor of *The Lancet* did not minimize the importance of Nunneley's charges, but fueled the flames of controversy by spurring on Lister's supporters: "Only experience can determine the actual value of carbolic acid; but Mr. Nunneley has fairly thrown down the gauntlet to those who advocated its use, and we trust that his challenge will not remain unanswered."[75] It did go unanswered by Lister himself for three weeks, probably because in the interim he changed posts, assuming the chair of surgery formerly occupied by his father-in-law in Edinburgh. There were other circumstances which must also have delayed his rebuttal. Syme had resigned because of illness and died the following June. The health of Lister's father was also failing, and he expired in only two months.[76]

Shortly before his death, Lister's father had shared a loving, spiritual perspective with his son, telling him that "however slowly & imperfectly the improvements suggested by thee may be adopted & however thy claims may be slighted or disputed, it is a great thing to *have been permitted to be the means of introducing so great a blessing as the antiseptic Treatment to thy fellow mortals.*" He concluded his remarks with the encourag-

---

[73] Thomas Nunneley, "Address in Surgery," *The British Medical Journal* (7 August 1869): 156; E. Gaskell, "Medical Literature," in *Medicine and Science in the 1860s*, ed. F. N. L. Poynter (London: Wellcome Institute for the History of Medicine, 1968), p. 308; Cartwright, "Antiseptic Surgery," p. 94.

[74] Nunneley, "Address," pp. 152, 155–56.

[75] James G. Wakley, "Mr. Nunneley on Carbolic Acid," *The Lancet* (14 August 1869): 245.

[76] James G. Wakley, "The Appointment of Mr. Lister," *The Lancet* (21 August 1869): 277; Fisher, *Joseph Lister*, pp. 167–68, 170, 176.

ing words that there was "abundant cause to persevere."[77] The elder Lister not only had faith in his son, but also in a higher purpose. He believed in "a time to heal."

When the younger Lister finally had time to respond to Nunneley, he exposed one inexcusable misstatement by him. He had been wrong when he asserted that the antiseptic method was not widely used in Leeds and that the surgeons there had lost faith in it. One of their number, T. Pridgin Teale, contradicted Nunneley in a note to Lister and gave Lister permission to publish it. Lister did so, along with a scathing opinion of Nunneley. "That he should dogmatically oppose a treatment which he so little understands; and which, by his own admission, he has never tried," wrote Lister, "is a matter of small moment."[78]

By this time, the editor of *The British Medical Journal,* the official publication of the British Medical Association, had become more concerned with stopping the personal attacks because they were overshadowing the issue. In spite of Lister's condescending attitude toward Nunneley, the editor blamed others for initiating a smear campaign. He absolved Lister, writing, "It is, we believe, chiefly from disciples, and not from himself, that strong statements have emanated." Clearly, this was not the case, but the editor wanted to extend the benefit of the doubt to the former Glasgow surgeon.[79]

This courteous treatment, however, was not necessary because Lister was not easily insulted and "was not afraid of offending people where principles were involved." What annoyed him the most was having to leave his experiments on the management of wounds to answer outrageous charges "that he was claiming to be the originator of the germ theory and even the discoverer of phenol." Certain of Lister's habits were also very upsetting to others. For example, he would not tell people what they owed him after he had treated them, but left it up to them to decide how much to pay. Also, once he accepted a case, the patient would not be returned to the family physician. One of the enemies Lister made was a fellow-surgeon, who "once lay in wait for him with a whip."[80]

Most of Lister's enemies were thankfully more subtle. D. Campbell Black, a surgeon from Glasgow, considered the use of carbolic acid futile and potentially harmful, if only in the public's perception. As a self-appointed spokesman for "the bulk of the profession in Glasgow," he denigrated it as "the latest toy of medical science so-called." Then, referring "to the carbolic acid mania," Black dismissed it as "a plausible theory, based on false premises, and bolstered up by coincidences." He further added,

> Medical men cannot be too cautious in mounting hobbies, or in being led away by the seductive influence of discovery. There is nothing more calculated to shake the faith of the public in our art—nothing more opposed to the true progress of scientific medicine or surgery.[81]

[77] Joseph Jackson Lister to Joseph Lister, 6 June 1869, Western Manuscripts, Wellcome Institute for the History of Medicine, London, MS 6965, 67.

[78] Joseph Lister, "Mr. Nunneley and the Antiseptic Treatment," *The British Medical Journal* (28 August 1869): 256–57.

[79] Jonathan Hutchinson, "Carbolic Acid Treatment of Wounds," *The British Medical Journal* (4 September 1869): 269–70.

[80] Edward Best, "Joseph Lister (1827–1912)," in *Mid-Nineteenth-Century Scientists,* ed. John North (Oxford: Pergamon Press, 1969), p. 147.

[81] D. Campbell Black, "Mr. Nunneley and the Antiseptic Treatment (Carbolic Acid)," *The British Medical Journal* (4 September 1869): 281.

The real purpose of Black's entry in *The British Medical Journal* was to defend Thomas Nunneley against Joseph Lister. He said he had heard no negative views expressed about Nunneley's address and tried to deflect Lister's rejoinder to Nunneley. Whereas Lister had questioned Nunneley's ability to grasp his ideas, Black answered that "if Mr. Nunneley has misapprehended, I wonder exceedingly who has apprehended the intricacies of this surgical arcanum." Certainly, according to Black, Thomas Keith, a pioneer in ovariotomy, had not understood Lister's system and was not one who washed his hands in carbolized oil or performed surgery "behind the antiseptic screen."[82]

Regrettably, Black was as given to error as the man he defended. Keith unreservedly attested to the value of antiseptics and revealed that he had incorporated them, in one form or another, in all of his surgeries. This was all the more amazing because he had performed ninety-two ovariotomies in Edinburgh since 1862, and they were considered the most hazardous of all operations due to the necessity of cutting through the abdomen. He credited Spencer Wells, another specialist in female maladies, with introducing him to "tar-bags," but for approximately three years he had also worked with carbolic acid. At the time his letter in response to Black was published, Keith was "invariably" subscribing to Lister's plan. He lamented Black's vindictiveness toward Lister, especially coming from a Glasgow physician "on the eve of his leaving" that city, and humbly added, "I think I am only now beginning to realise what Mr. Lister's antiseptic method and his carbolised animal-ligatures are yet to do for surgery."[83]

Black could not resist the opportunity to reiterate his views in a letter to *The Lancet* responding to Keith's assault. He opined that "the soaking of sponges in, [and] the smearing of instruments and fingers with, carbolic acid, and carbolic acid drapery, to say the least of the practice, seems to me frivolous and unscientific." Again, Black could not fathom "this carbolic-acid fuss" and scorned the amount of time that was being wasted "in unlearning." The most damaging element in his correspondence, though, came from statistics he had gleaned from the *Medical Times and Gazette* which showed that there had been essentially no change in death rates from amputations and compound fractures at the Glasgow Royal Infirmary between 1860 and 1868. From 1860 to 1862, one-third of all amputees died, while around one-fourth of patients with compound fractures died. The figures for 1867 and 1868, when Lister's system was introduced, showed that more than a third of the amputees still perished, and that in 1868, "a year in which . . . all the surgeons to the hospital used carbolic acid," the same was true in cases of compound fracture, Lister's showpiece.[84] Obviously, Black's reiteration of these figures caused the glow of the antiseptic system to dim for many.

Word of the mortality comparisons also reached France in a publication entitled *Bulletin General de Therapeutique Medicale et Chirurgicale*. According to Edward H. Bennett, who was citing an article from the French periodical in *The Dublin Journal of Medical Science,* the number of deaths since the advent of carbolic acid "has been

---

[82] Ibid.
[83] Keith started using tar-bags on his twelfth ovariotomy, after having tried bags of charcoal, sulphite of soda, and sulphate of iron. Thomas Keith, "Antiseptic Treatment," *The British Medical Journal* (18 September 1869): 335–36.
[84] Donald Campbell Black, "Antiseptic Treatment," *The Lancet* (9 October 1869): 524–25.

greater in Mr. Lister's hospital . . . than it was some years ago before it was known." It also claimed that Continental physicians had less respect for Lister's chosen antiseptic than British practitioners and that "it obtains these marvellous properties, above all, in the hands of English surgeons, who are infatuated with it."[85]

Another Irish practitioner, however, who authored an article for the same issue in which Bennett's report appeared, said that the antiseptic principle "leaves little to be desired as regards the treatment of wounds" and that his surgical department "would seem almost to have attained by these means the highest degree of perfection of which it is capable." In his closing remarks, he predicted that Lister's "plan of treatment" would undoubtedly "gain a lasting reputation for its author."[86] What was true of his department of surgery was also true of Lister's wards, but other wards of the Glasgow Royal Infirmary did not follow the antiseptic pattern, at least not with any consistency. In a pseudonymous letter to *The Lancet,* Lister's wards were described as having a "fresh, healthy atmosphere" and an "absence of any smell," as opposed to "those wards which are not under his care, and where the treatment is not so accurately or not at all carried out."[87] This contrast temporarily explained the infirmary's overall mortality percentages for the 1860s but did not provide the statistics that were necessary to distinguish Lister's successes from the results of the other surgeons, whether they had tried carbolic acid or not. Lister determined to correct this oversight in the coming year.

---

[85] Edward H. Bennett, "Report on Surgery," *The Dublin Journal of Medical Science* 48 (August 1869): 181.

[86] Robert M'Donnell, "Observations on Traumatic Fever and the Treatment of Wounds by the Antiseptic Method," *The Dublin Journal of Medical Science* 48 (August 1869): 42–43, 45.

[87] Practitioner [pseud.], "Mr. Lister's Antiseptic Treatment," *The Lancet* (30 October 1869): 629.

4. National Competition as a Factor in the Diffusion of Listerism

With the dawning of a new decade and without his father to temper his responses, Lister no longer remained content merely to defend his system but mounted a campaign to justify himself. He returned to the fray with a vengeance on New Year's Day, 1870. In an article for *The Lancet* entitled "On the Effects of the Antiseptic System of Treatment upon the Salubrity of a Surgical Hospital," Lister exhibited a stunning lack of tact and a certain degree of conceit. His egotism was obvious when he boasted that a "striking change" had occurred in his wards, "converting them from some of the most unhealthy in the kingdom into models of healthiness."[1] He also prophesied that "whether in the form which it has now reached, or in some other and more perfect shape," his method would enjoy "universal adoption." His bluntness manifested itself when he blamed the administrators of the Glasgow Royal Infirmary for worsening death rates, and he interspersed injudicious criticisms of them throughout the article. Lister attacked the superintendent for not having cleaned his wards during the past three years, a decision the superintendent made because he could not find enough visible dirt to justify the expense.[2] Lister also accused "the managing body," with which he claimed to be "engaged in a perpetual contest," of filling the hospital beyond capacity. Lister was staunchly opposed to their actions and thought it was

> fairly attributable to the firmness of my resistance in this matter that, though my patients suffered from the evils alluded to in a way that was sickening and often heartrending, so as to make me sometimes feel it a questionable privilege to be connected with the institution, yet none of my wards ever assumed the frightful condition which sometimes showed itself in other parts of the building, making it necessary to shut them up entirely for a time.[3]

Lister's main purpose, though, was to refute the charges that had been made regarding death rates in his wards. He compared the figures from 1867 to 1869 to those from 1864 and 1866; figures for 1865 were incomplete. Sixteen of thirty-five amputees had died before carbolic acid was used, while only six of forty expired afterward.[4] The impact of these numbers motivated the editor of *The Lancet* to call upon London hospitals a second time to "fairly and crucially" test Lister's method. He suggested that some of Lister's students should be stationed in "a surgical ward . . . known for its unhealthiness" to oversee the experiment properly, deducing that what had been achieved in Glasgow "ought to be procurable in London."[5]

---

[1] Joseph Lister, "On the Effects of the Antiseptic System of Treatment upon the Salubrity of a Surgical Hospital," *The Lancet* (1 January 1870): 4.
[2] Ibid., (8 January 1870): 42.
[3] Ibid., (1 January 1870): 4.
[4] Ibid., (8 January 1870): 40.
[5] James G. Wakley, "Hospitalism and the Antiseptic System," *The Lancet* (15 January 1870): 91.

Wakley's editorial on the antiseptic system also contained comments on "hospitalism," the rampant diseases caused by cross-infection which prompted James Y. Simpson to campaign for the destruction of certain medical facilities. In essence, Wakley presented *The Lancet*'s readers with two alternatives, demolish hospitals or pattern wards after those of Lister.[6] Undoubtedly, health care providers contributed to the problem of nosocomial infections as they spread disease by going directly from patient to patient, or by tending to the living immediately after doing autopsies and dissections, without even washing their hands. The introduction of large numbers of medical students into teaching hospitals added to the difficulty, and the "selective development of virulent strains of microorganisms by rapid and repeated human transference could also have played a part."[7]

The administrators of the Glasgow Royal Infirmary naturally replied to Lister's article on the healthfulness of their facility. (See Figure 7.) They denied Lister's accusations and refused to acknowledge that they had either admitted too many patients or been guilty of cleaning his wards less often than the others. As far as an ongoing disagreement with Lister was concerned, they recalled only one, and it was over the fact that he kept his patients too long and only saw two-thirds as many as the other surgeons. In their estimation, Lister's innovations had not been particularly significant. Instead, they took credit themselves for any improvements that had come about, claiming that

> the improved health and satisfactory condition of the hospital, which has been as marked in the medical as in the surgical department, is mainly attributable to the better ventilation, the improved dietary, and the excellent nursing to which the Directors have given so much attention of late years.[8]

Lister could not let these comments pass without a rebuttal and wrote that crediting airflow, food, and the staff with the improved condition of his wards was "simply out of the question." He even affirmed his belief that the secretary for the administration, who wrote the letter, had taken it upon himself to attribute the hospital's success to such factors. He did express regret at having used the word "contest" to describe his difference of opinion with the directors, but he rejected their complaint that because he did not treat as many patients as other surgeons he was inefficient. His wards did not have private rooms or additional beds like most others. From his vantage point, he had humiliated himself, to some extent, by publishing mortality totals for 1864 and 1866. He also felt that the managers should have looked upon his success as theirs.[9]

Many years later, however, when another facility was being built for the Glasgow

---

[6] Ibid; S. Selwyn, "Sir James Simpson and Hospital Cross-Infection," *Medical History* 9 (July 1965): 242–45.

[7] Edward D. Churchill, "The Pandemic of Wound Infection in Hospitals: Studies in the History of Wound Healing," *Journal of the History of Medicine and Allied Sciences* 20 (October 1965): 401; for a good discussion of the status of hospitalism or nosocomial infections today, see Lois Magner, *A History of Medicine* (New York: Marcel Dekker, Inc., 1992), pp. 301–302.

[8] Henry Lamond, "Professor Lister and the Glasgow Infirmary," *The Lancet* (29 January 1870): 175; for the analysis of one who has studied the statistics from the Glasgow Royal Infirmary in the 1800s and agrees more with the assessment of the managers than with Lister, see David Hamilton, "The Nineteenth-Century Surgical Revolution—Antisepsis or Better Nutrition?," *Bulletin of the History of Medicine* 56 (Spring 1982): 37–40.

[9] Joseph Lister, "The Glasgow Infirmary and the Antiseptic Treatment," *The Lancet* (5 February 1870): 210–11.

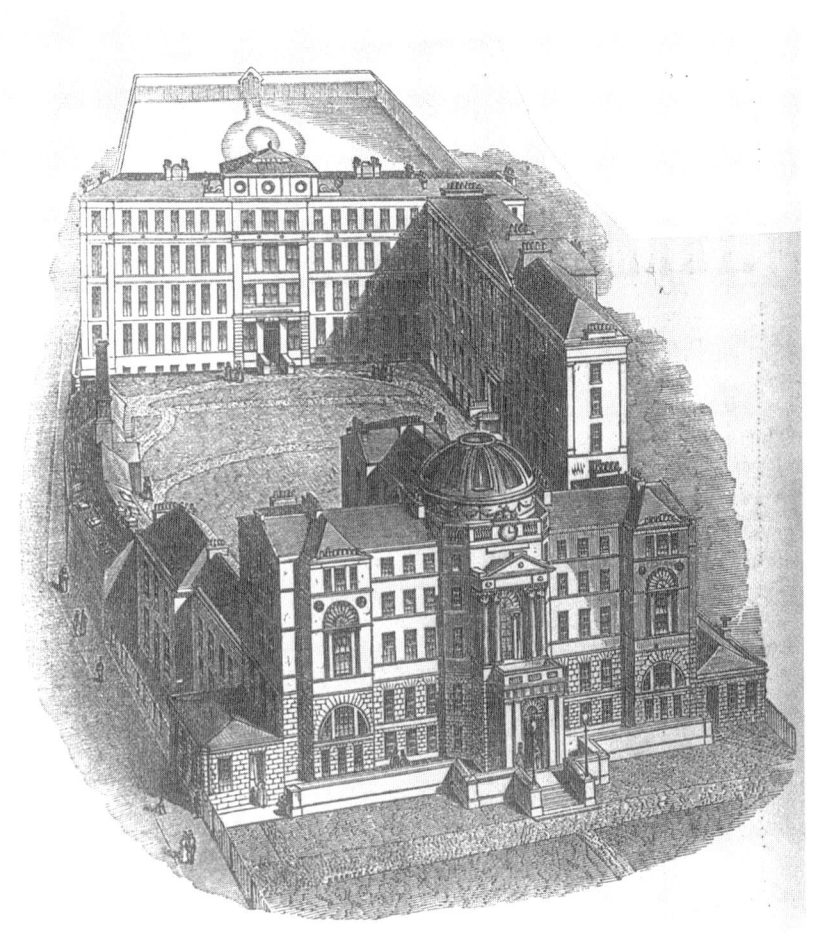

Figure 7. Glasgow Royal Infirmary

Royal Infirmary, Lister wrote that he "could not honestly say that the old surgical was unhealthy. Its system of ventilation was admirable." Nevertheless, he did "not doubt" that if the proposed structure had only one surgeon per ward, each with its own nurses, it would "be an improvement on the old, but more as to being more *commodious* than more salubrious."[10] No matter how efficient the system of ventilation was, studies have shown that more air is not the answer and can even be detrimental. It is clean air that expedites healing.[11]

The infirmary's administrators soon found support for their position from one of the physicians who had worked in Glasgow while Lister was there. James Morton,

---

[10] Joseph Lister to Hector Clare Cameron, 20 January 1908, Joseph Lister Papers, Library, Royal College of Surgeons of Edinburgh, Edinburgh, GD5, 90.
[11] O. M. Lidwell, "Joseph Lister and Infection from the Air," *Epidemiology and Infection* 99 (1987): 573–76.

whose eight-year tenure had ended in October, 1867, assessed the value of carbolic acid and concluded that it "was certainly not superior, barely equal, to some of the other antiseptics in common use."[12] In fact, he quibbled with the designation "The Antiseptic System," alleging that Lister's technique should instead be called "an antiseptic mode of dressing." Morton also quickly dismissed the germ theory. He stated that it "has not been satisfactorily established" and disputed the contention that the air carries dangerous organisms. "It is a fearful idea," he reasoned,

> [and] fortunately, for thousands, a baseless theory—that there are formations in nature, and actually floating in the air, which are constantly in readiness to aid the grim king in his onslaughts upon frail humanity. Our human nature shudders at the thought. It certainly is not an "air from heaven;" and may, without hyperbole, be styled a "blast from hell." . . . Nature is here regarded as some murderous hag . . . whose fiendish machinations must be counteracted. She must be entrapped into good behavior; she is no longer to be trusted.[13]

Six months after the exchange concerning the Glasgow Royal Infirmary, Lister submitted an article to *The Lancet* describing the condition of his wards in Edinburgh. He reported no pyemia or hospital gangrene, but did admit having two cases of erysipelas, which he blamed on external causes. They both had happened the previous December, and Lister thought that they were caused by exposure to cold. Primarily, Lister used the article to pass on a letter from a noted Danish surgeon, M. H. Saxtorph, who verified that there was no pyemia in his wards either and that all of his amputees had survived since his adoption of the antiseptic method after a visit to Scotland the previous year. Armed with Saxtorph's testimony Lister took aim at the surgeons of London. Assailing their sense of national superiority, he goaded, "It may seem strange that results like these should have been obtained in Copenhagen, when so little approach to them has yet been made in the capital of England."[14]

Lister did not think that his system's lack of success in London was due to too few trials. Instead, he blamed it on more fundamental failings. London surgeons were too preoccupied with his choice of carbolic acid as an antiseptic, they refused to accept the germ theory, and they were careless in carrying out the procedures required by his method. In short, Lister thought that London surgeons were lazy because of their unwillingness to consider new ideas and sloppy in their technical skills. He assured his readers that his results were not due "to some specific virtue in the agent," that he "should expect" failure by "those who doubt or disbelieve" Pasteur, and that surgeons professing to imitate his technique would "throw up the attempt in disgust" unless they meticulously duplicated every detail until it "has become habitual and instinctive."[15] The editor of *The Lancet* summarized the problem in London best when he

---

[12] James Morton, "Carbolic Acid: Its Therapeutic Position, with Special Reference to its Use in Severe Surgical Cases," *The Lancet* (5 February 1870): 188.
[13] Ibid., (29 January 1870): 155–56.
[14] Joseph Lister, "Further Evidence Regarding the Effects of the Antiseptic System of Treatment upon the Salubrity of a Surgical Hospital," *The Lancet* (27 August 1870): 287–88.
[15] Ibid.

observed that "the incredulity of leading English surgeons is so general" but that the accomplishments of men like "Lister, Saxtorph, and others are new facts in surgery, or rather physiology, and must have a scientific definition."[16]

In 1870 Lister found another opportunity to extend his system to the Continent. Both the French and the Germans asked him "to furnish some rules for the antiseptic treatment of wounded soldiers," who were casualties of the Franco-Prussian War.[17] Although his guidelines were not received early enough to substantially reduce battle-field deaths, more surgeons on the Continent did become aware of Lister's methods. This was especially the case with the Prussians, who used carbolic acid in their hospitals and ambulances.[18] Coincidentally, William MacCormac, the Belfast surgeon who had earlier endorsed Lister's system, treated the wounded at Sedan, where amputees fared particularly well and where such ailments as erysipelas and gangrene seldom occurred. Pyemia, on the other hand, was "common," but if anything, that fact refuted the tenets of hospitalism, which attributed the sickness to poor ventilation and over-crowding. During the Franco-Prussian War, wounded troops were often treated in the open or in small numbers at private dwellings.[19]

At the meeting of the Medical Society of London on October 17, 1870, the pre-siding officer called attention to a report in *The Times* concerning the beneficial aspects of open-air surgery practiced on the battlefields of France. In his opinion, there were "many elements of truth in the observations that have been made . . . with regard to the active part that these germs take in determining unhealthy processes in a wound." He went on to say that Lister's "facts have been open to observation, and have not, it would appear, been impugned."[20] Not all members of the medical profession in England's capital hesitated to use words like "truth" and "facts" when talking about the germ theory and the antiseptic principle.

It must be remembered that at this time those who used the word "germ" to de-scribe an agent of infection branded themselves as adherents of the germ theory. Wakley refused to use the term in *The Lancet* and chose instead to write about "septic elements contained in the air."[21] Lawson Tait, a Birmingham surgeon who later be-came famous for his aseptic technique in abdominal operations, agreed with Wakley and listed six instances in which he "carried out most faithfully" the antiseptic system. Carbolic acid either did no good or "delayed the healing," while three other cases handled with no disinfectants at all "got well without any suppuration." Tait catego-rized germs as "supposititious" and wrote that "despite the most persevering and hon-est trials," the merits of antisepsis "have been greatly over-rated, and its good results, which are quite as uncertain as those of other means, are due more to the greater care taken of the cases, and to the exclusion of air."[22] Tait had studied at the feet of Lister's

[16] James G. Wakley, "The Antiseptic Principle in Surgery," *The Lancet* (17 September 1870): 411.
[17] Joseph Lister, "A Method of Antiseptic Treatment Applicable to Wounded Soldiers in the Present War," *The British Medical Journal* (3 September 1870): 243–44.
[18] James G. Wakley, "A Sanitary Detachment on the Battle-Field," *The Lancet* (1 October 1870): 481.
[19] James G. Wakley, "The Wounded About Sedan," *The Lancet* (8 October 1870): 517.
[20] James G. Wakley, "Medical Society of London," *The Lancet* (29 October 1870): 604–605.
[21] James G. Wakley, "Antiseptic Surgery," *The Lancet* (29 October 1870): 613.
[22] Lawson Tait, "Cases Treated Antiseptically on Lister's Method," *The Lancet* (14 January 1871): 45–46.

early enemy, Simpson, who held that cures could be effected by removing patients from miasmatic environs. Simpson died in 1870, and his former pupil took up the gauntlet against Lister in January of the following year.[23]

London surgeons also responded to Lister's challenge, and new reports from various hospitals in the metropolis on the usefulness of the antiseptic method began to appear again in *The Lancet*. Apparently, many London hospitals had abandoned the use of carbolic acid after early uses in 1868 and 1869. Wakley prefaced these reports with an analysis of what had transpired since the last flurry of notices. In its earliest trials, carbolic acid

> was very generally applied in some form or other, and under various conditions; and the practice of those hospitals in which the experiment was made with earnestness sufficient to afford reliable data appeared to encourage a persistence in the careful and studious application of the system. It appears, however, that in many of the hospitals this subject has not survived that first glow of interest which a new thing rarely fails to kindle.[24]

From the renewed tests conducted in 1871, though, it is clear that some London hospitals experienced greater success with the antiseptic method the second time around. At St. George's Hospital, for example, Lister's practice saw "such marked results as to raise it high in the esteem and confidence of the hospital staff." This was most noticeable in the treatment of abscesses, the medical problem singled out by Lawson Tait as the least suited to carbolic acid. Zinc chloride was considered as advantageous as carbolic acid at Middlesex Hospital, though "good results" had been obtained using the latter. The third and last of the initial wave of new entries from the capital of England was that from London Hospital. Nearly fifty surgical procedures performed since the fall of 1869 were, for the most part, "conspicuous for the small amount of constitutional disturbance produced by very severe injuries." After only "a few days" of treatment, patients were "free from pain," and "they ate and slept well." They also "had an appearance of health by no means usual after extensive wounds."[25]

Immediately following these reports from London was a series of examples from the records of Bennet May, house-surgeon at Birmingham General Hospital. Coming only two pages after Tait's tirade, and from the same city, they revealed that some surgeons had enough success with carbolic acid to regularly administer it. Yet, the results were not sufficiently convincing to commend Lister's system as exemplary. None of the wounds produced true pus, which was an odorous discharge, but a third of them were ultimately healed through ordinary means when recovery from carbolic-acid dressings proved too difficult or too slow. Two cases turned for the worse, one "possibly from admission of air" and the other from a "typhoid condition."[26]

The experiences of another metropolitan institution, St. Mary's Hospital, were

[23] J. Duns, *Memoir of Sir James Y. Simpson, Bart.* (Edinburgh: Edmonston and Douglas, 1873), pp. 511, 520–21, 526–31.

[24] James G. Wakley, "A Mirror of the Practice of Medicine and Surgery in the Hospitals of London," *The Lancet* (14 January 1871): 47.

[25] Ibid., pp. 47–48.

[26] James G. Wakley, "Provincial Hospital Reports," *The Lancet* (14 January 1871): 48–49.

described in *The Lancet* on the first of April. Its correspondent was Bernard O'Connor, who six months earlier had presented a paper on the antiseptic treatment of wounds at a meeting of the hospital's Medical Society. Now, he was acting as dresser for one of the surgeons and outlined the course of four subjects whose injuries were managed antiseptically. Some discharge occurred with two of them, but one was from a previous operation in the summer of 1870, and the other was due to a dressing slipping off. O'Connor had "acquired the theory and art of the carbolic-acid treatment under the personal tuition of Professor Lister," and it showed. St. Mary's Hospital had accepted the challenge to hire someone who had studied the technique firsthand and witnessed conclusive evidence of the feasibility of the antiseptic principle.[27]

What O'Connor had seen with his own eyes were a new dressing, antiseptically treated rubber tubes for drainage, and a sprayer to saturate the operating room with carbolic acid. The new dressing consisted of eight gauze layers with a strip of mackintosh between the two that were farthest away from the wound; mackintosh is a rubberized cloth that was inserted to stop air from contacting the secretions, which provided a fluid route for germs to enter the patient. The drainage tubes were steeped in carbolic acid before being used and insured that any suppuration caused by the caustic agent itself escaped. The spray was a one-percent solution for preventing germs from invading the body, especially when dressings were changed. Lister had tried a one to forty spray solution earlier, but it had irritated his hands and lungs.

One historian has noted that many considered 1871 to be "the beginning of antisepsis proper" because the spray showed more abundantly the importance of accepting the germ theory. Lindsay Granshaw of London's Wellcome Institute for the History of Medicine has convincingly explained this perception of a watershed by asserting, "While the application of carbolic acid could be seen as little different from applying some new specific, the spray, which had no contact with the wound, could not. It became a symbol of faith in the existence of germs, as airborne causes of disease."[28]

The spray became a symbol of ridicule, too, especially when the original atomizer gave way to "The Donkey Engine," a sprayer also worked by hand but positioned on a tall tripod. (See Figure 8.) This was eventually replaced by a steam machine, which was much smaller and very mobile. Lister's assistants took turns laboring with the early versions of the sprayer, and some of them had to stop helping him because of sensitivity to carbolic acid. Patients were also irritated by the spray, the most famous being Queen Victoria. During her surgery Lister was aided by William Jenner, who misdirected the vapor and got fumes in her eyes. When she "complained, Jenner excused himself by saying that he was 'only the man who worked the bellows.'" This case was serious, and the blunder caused additional concern, but Lister was always solemn when he operated. Usually, he "was followed in procession by his train of

---

[27] O'Connor had toured Lister's wards in Edinburgh, leaving them as "an earnest admirer," and had been recommended to the London medical establishment as one who was "conversant with all the details of the method" inaugurated by Lister; he was promoted in the hope that he would give the antiseptic technique its definitive test in England's capital. James G. Wakley, "St. Mary's Hospital," *The Lancet* (1 April 1871): 446–47; Wakley, "Antiseptic Surgery," (29 October 1870): 613.

[28] Lindsay Granshaw, "'Upon this Principle I have based a Practice': The Development and Reception of Antisepsis in Britain, 1867–90," in *Medical Innovations in Historical Perspective,* ed. John V. Pickstone (New York: St. Martin's Press, 1992), pp. 27–29.

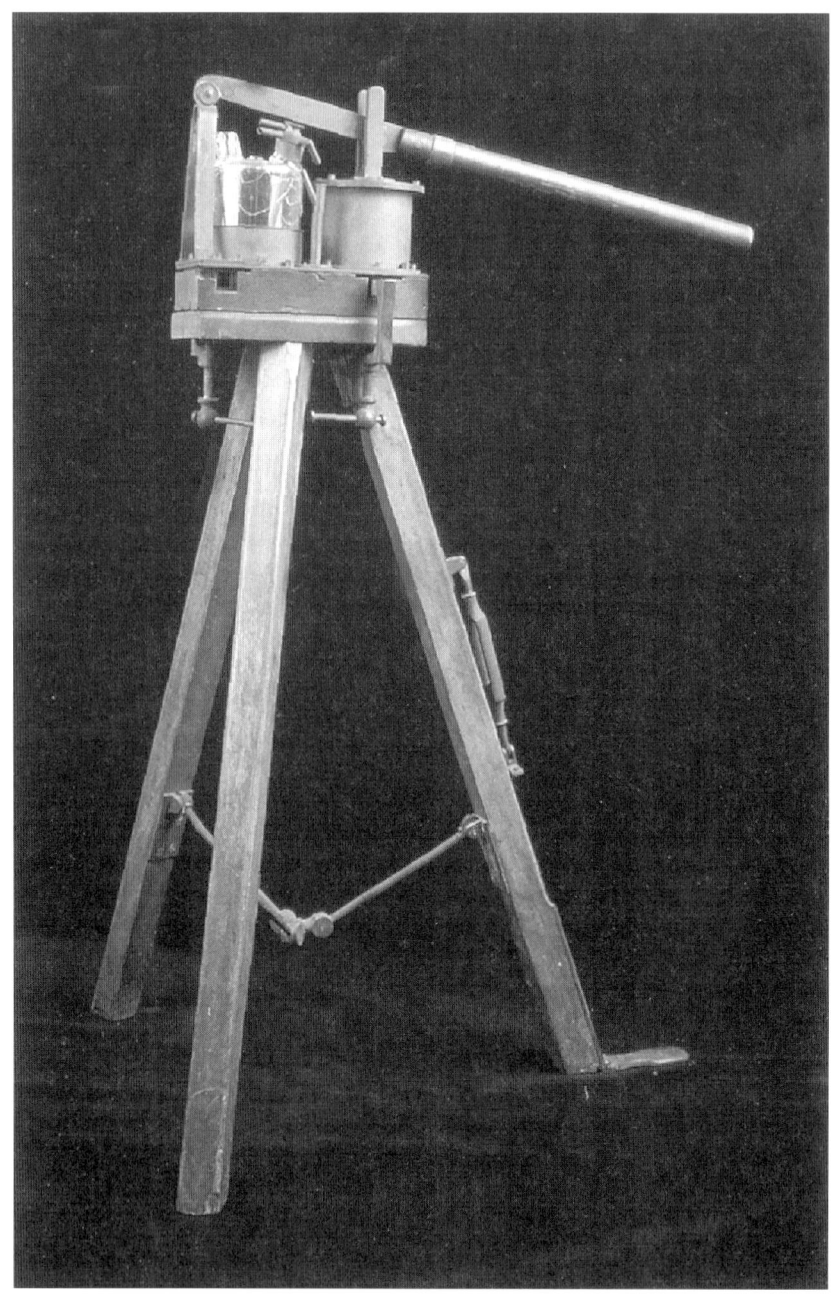

Figure 8. Donkey Engine

dressers, the first of whom bore aloft the sacred spray. Once the silence was broken by some ribald student whose voice was heard intoning, 'Let us spray.'"[29]

Two months after O'Connor's report, Lister spoke at a convention of the Edinburgh Medico-Chirurgical Society, where he personally described the improvements he had made in his method. He announced that the antiseptic gauze was taking the place of lac plaster because it was more absorbent and clung to the skin better. Lac, a resinous substance found in southern Asia, is used in producing varnish and sealing wax. Lister had been mixing it with plaster of Paris to make an antiseptic covering for wounds. The gauze, however, consisted of "carbolic acid stored in insoluble resin among the fibres, with the addition of paraffin to avoid undue adhesiveness, in the proportions of one part of carbolic acid, five parts of resin, and seven parts of paraffin." With an exaggerated tone, Lister anticipated those who might reject this covering on the grounds that it blocked needed access to the air. Eagerly preempting them, he said,

> While speaking of the advantages of the gauze, there is one other to which I cannot forbear alluding. If you apply this mass of it, consisting of thirty-two layers, closely to the face, you find you can breathe freely through it, as through a respirator. Hence, Sir, one great advantage of this dressing will be, that it will deprive those who discuss the antiseptic treatment of all excuse for speaking of it as operating by "excluding the air." We do not exclude the gases of the atmosphere at all, but adopt efficient means to destroy the energy of its floating ferments.[30]

The phrase in quotation marks was an obvious attack on Lawson Tait, whose criticisms from six months earlier were still vivid in Lister's memory.

The inability to forget personal affronts engendered a certain amount of self-consciousness and defensiveness in Lister and inspired him to use a variety of rhetorical devices to bring his enemies to bay. On August 10, 1871, he had his first opportunity to speak to the entire medical community of the United Kingdom. He delivered the surgical address at the thirty-ninth annual meeting of the British Medical Association, which convened in Plymouth. First, he linked criticism of him with possible impediment of his system's progress. After boldly announcing that his method was "calculated . . . to revolutionize almost every department of surgical practice," he modestly confessed, "The fact that my name is associated with this topic tended to make me shrink from such a course." Lister then shifted emotions again and tried to move his audience from feelings of pity to embarrassment. He started by discussing the way his countrymen had castigated Pasteur, which, of course, was an attack on those who opposed the germ theory. Lister first described Pasteur's experiment with urine, "a putrescible liquid" which did not change when it was boiled "in a flask with an attenuated and contorted neck."[31]

---

[29] Hector Charles Cameron, *Joseph Lister: The Friend of Man* (London: William Heinemann, 1949), pp. 88–89; Rickman John Godlee, *Lord Lister,* 3d ed. (Oxford: The Clarendon Press, 1924), pp. 305–306.
[30] Joseph Lister, "On Some Cases Illustrating the Results of Excision of the Wrist for Caries, the Treatment of Deformity from Contracted Cicatrix, and Antiseptic Dressing under Circumstances of Difficulty, Including Amputation at the Hip-Joint," *Edinburgh Medical Journal* 17 (August 1871): 147, 150.
[31] Joseph Lister, *The Collected Papers,* 2 vols. (Oxford: The Clarendon Press, 1909), 2:172–73.

Again targeting certain British physicians who remained unnamed but were recognized by all present, Lister shamefully acknowledged that he was "ready to blush for the character of our profession for scientific accuracy" and was "tempted to doubt whether some of the commentators can have enjoyed the advantages of sufficient education either in chemical physics or in logic." He followed this gratuitous insult by an effort to separate antiseptic surgery from the germ theory. To encourage more surgeons to try his method, Lister swallowed his pride and said,

> I do not ask you to believe that the septic particles are organisms. That they are self-propagating, like living beings, and that their energy is extinguished by precisely the same agencies as extinguish vitality, such as heat and the various chemical substances to which I have referred, is certain, and is of the utmost practical importance. . . . Nor do I enter upon the question whether spontaneous generation can take place at the present day upon the surface of our globe. To do this, would be to engage in doubtful disputations, which I promised to avoid.[32]

One final characteristic of Lister's presentation was its theatricality. Although he had "greatly exceeded" the length assigned for his talk, he further imposed on his captive audience by accusing surgeons "in many quarters" of "apathy." To jolt them out of their complacency, he quoted from *Macbeth,* in which Shakespeare wrote,

> Can such things be,
> And overcome us like a summer's cloud
> Without our special wonder?[33]

Indeed, one wonders whether Lister's condescending attitude toward the London medical establishment aided or hindered his cause. Hindsight seems to indicate that his willingness to personalize the debate impeded the adoption of antisepsis.

Almost in spite of Lister, adherents to his technique did multiply. An unexpected boost was furnished by A. Ernest Sansom, physician to both the Royal Hospital for Diseases of the Chest and the North-Eastern Hospital for Children in London. He authored the first full-length book on the antiseptic system, which appeared in 1871. Sansom described the use of carbolic acid as "very general," subsequent to Lister's popularization of it, but did not leave out the fact that there had been "apparent discrepancy in individual experience" due to a lack of knowledge "of the chemical characteristics and the pathological influence of the agent." Finding that carbolic acid was "singularly destitute of any direct chemical power," he nevertheless purported that "the chemical properties of a body are in no direct relation whatever with the power of that body to arrest fermentive or putrefactive changes." What was pertinent to its strength was whether it was used to disinfect water or air. Employed for the former, it was less powerful than numerous other disinfectants, but its utility for the latter was supreme

---

[32] Ibid., 2:175, 178.
[33] Ibid., 2:197.

among antiseptics. Sansom equated disinfectants and antiseptics but tagged those agents that only dispel scents as "deodorants."[34]

Sansom did not, however, consider "the carbolic acid method of treatment" and "the antiseptic method of treatment" to be one and the same. Realizing that Lister had been hailed "as the champion of carbolic acid," he countered with, "I am sure the inference of those who thus style him is a false one. In his practice Professor Lister employs many antiseptics besides carbolic acid as the chief." Sansom did view putrefaction and fermentation as "analogous" processes and, thus, openly embraced the germ theory of disease, although he leaned toward the interpretation "that the active agents in inducing the changes are vegetable, not animal, structures."[35]

Sansom's researches were, by his own admission, in a stage of infancy, but other surgeons, like Charles Roberts, respected them as "carefully investigated." Roberts, who was also employed at an institution for young people, the Victoria Hospital for Children, had little respect for Lister, though. He ascribed the origin of the antiseptic system, not just the first use of carbolic acid, to others and complained that "Mr. Lister's complicated practice has retarded rather than advanced its development." Ostensibly, Roberts wrote in such a disparaging fashion because he thought that more had been claimed for carbolic acid than it was able to produce, and he attacked those who claimed that it could kill "the gaseous and liquid products of decomposition" after putrefaction had already begun. Reading more closely, however, one sees that he vehemently deplored its application to "young epithelium," a practice continued by many physicians after Lister had declared that it was "injurious."[36]

These grave objections were carried in an April, 1872, installment of *The Lancet.* Eight months had come and gone since Lister's address in Plymouth, but Charles Roberts was clearly ignorant of the speech. Lister had already qualified the effects of carbolic acid, stating that it "is always injurious in its own action; a necessary evil, incurred to attain a greater good. To suppose that it is useful by its own operation in some specific manner unknown to us, is an entire mistake."[37] According to Richard B. Fisher, the article by Roberts was the sole entry on the antiseptic system in *The Lancet* for the entire year. Lister and his followers interpreted the silence as irresponsibility, not consent. Fisher speculates that the relative quiet reflected a wait-and-see attitude by those who wanted more verification of Lister's method.[38]

Further evidence in support of the antiseptic technique appeared in the spring of 1873. William Haydon, a rural surgeon from the county of Devon, in which Plymouth is located, proffered an explanation for the shortfalls experienced by some who endeavored to appropriate Lister's system. He wrote that failure was often due to leaving part of the antiseptic method undone through oversight. Surgeons might omit the one step of Lister's technique that would turn out to be the determining factor in whether or not a wound healed. Haydon also identified many of those who refused to attempt the antiseptic method as "engaged in a country practice." They were leery of

[34] Arthur Ernest Sansom, *The Antiseptic System: A Treatise on Carbolic Acid and Its Compounds* (Philadelphia: J. B. Lippincott and Co., 1871), pp. 4, 200–201, 207–208.
[35] Ibid., pp. 250, 111–13.
[36] Charles Roberts, "The Action and Use of Antiseptics in Surgical Practice," *The Lancet* (27 April 1872): 570–71.
[37] Lister, *The Collected Papers,* 2:181.
[38] Richard B. Fisher, *Joseph Lister, 1827–1912* (New York: Stein and Day, 1977), p. 179.

the amount of time required, but also of the quality of care their patients would receive between "cottage" visits. He assured them that carbolic-acid dressings only had to be changed every three days instead of daily, that family members would not have to do anything in the interim, and that the patients would suffer less because of the sedative property of the antiseptic.[39]

An urban surgeon, Lister's nephew, also attested to the benefits of the antiseptic method. Rickman J. Godlee was surgical registrar at University College Hospital, and he proudly avowed that "the vital importance in surgery of the antiseptic system is now very generally recognised." He got permission to divulge the fact that his uncle incorporated boric acid and zinc chloride as antiseptics in certain types of injuries; the former was "invaluable" for "superficial sores" because of "its extreme blandness," and the latter was "remarkable" as "a most efficient corrector of putrefaction . . . preserving or pickling the part to which it is applied."[40] In other words, zinc chloride would be employed in cases where decomposition had started beforehand. Both of these agents were used sparingly by Lister, though, because they were not volatile like carbolic acid. In addition to the newsworthiness of Godlee's account, he demystified Lister's practice by making it known that

> it is a great mistake to suppose that in none of Mr. Lister's cases does suppuration occur, and still greater for any surgeon to relinquish the antiseptic treatment of a wound the moment a speck of pus appears in it. Mr. Lister lays great stress on the fact that suppuration may be caused by any abnormal stimulus whatever, whether the indirect or nervous, as in ordinary inflammation, or by the direct action of a chemical irritant, the latter class including that which results from the stimulation of an antiseptic salt as well as that which is caused by the products of putrefaction. It is obvious that it is the occurrence of putrefactive suppuration alone that involves the failure of the antiseptic treatment.[41]

If Lister's principle was crucial to the improvement of surgery, its significance was lost on John Wood, who delivered the address in surgery at the yearly gathering of the British Medical Association in August, 1873. The assembly convened in London, where many members of the medical profession were still intransigent with regard to the antiseptic plan. Wood's own track record with the technique showed a backward trend; in the fall of 1867 he had enjoyed substantial success, but a little more than a year later his results were mixed. Even when his results had been less than anticipated, he associated the failures with the poor hygiene of the hospital and continued to uphold carbolic acid as the best substance for producing a protective crust on wounds.[42]

---

[39] William Haydon, "On the Antiseptic Plan of Treatment," *Edinburgh Medical Journal* 18 (March 1873): 792; for the views of one hospital manager, who collected two sets of statistics on amputations from sixty-one and forty-four cottage hospitals, respectively, and concluded that their mortality rates were generally less than metropolitan hospitals, though both enjoyed equally good results with antisepsis, see Henry C. Burdett, "The Relative Mortality, after Amputations, of Large and Small Hospitals, and the Influence of the Antiseptic (Listerian) System upon such Mortality," *Journal of the Statistical Society* 45 (September 1882): 444–45, 451, 469, 472–73, 475.

[40] Rickman J. Godlee, "On the Antiseptic System," *The Lancet* (17 May 1873): 694–95.

[41] Ibid., (24 May 1873): 729.

[42] John Wood, "The Address in Surgery," *The Lancet* (9 August 1873): 182.

By the time of the Association's forty-first annual meeting, though, Wood was unimpressed with carbolic acid because it often did not promote healing or did so too slowly. In the adjacent wards of William Fergusson, who did not use antiseptics, the death toll was not noticeably higher. Fergusson has been called the "greatest operator at the middle of the century." He was particularly effective in dealing with cleft palate and harelip. "Out of 134 cases of cleft palate upon which he operated between 1828 and 1864 he was able to claim 129 successes, and among 400 cases of harelip operated upon by him during the same period there were only three failures." He invented such medical devices as the lion forceps, mouth gag, and speculum. He was also the one who had coined the term "conservative surgery." The stench of Fergusson's wards was worse than Wood's side, which the former "shrewdly attributed to the carbolic smell overpowering all others." As a result of Fergusson's comparable success, Wood decided

> that cases of recovery frequently occur under other methods, or no methods, and
> that at least as much depends upon the age and reparative power of the patient,
> the amount of blood poison formed or absorbed, and the general conditions
> of the atmosphere, as upon any system of treatment whatever.[43]

In what seemed to be poetic justice, Lister was hired by King's College Hospital after Fergusson's death four years later. At that time Lister expressed his strong personal opinion of Fergusson in a private letter describing how their teaching philosophies differed. Writing to an associate in Edinburgh in unsympathetic and scathing words, he pronounced, "The mere fact of Fergusson having held the clinical chair is surely a matter of no great moment; more especially as I should propose to hold the office not in a merely nominal manner as Sir William did, but as a place of downright hard work." Lister also told his colleague that another goal of his was to effect "the thorough working of the antiseptic system with a view to its diffusion in the Metropolis."[44]

Meanwhile, Joseph Lister contended that his energies to completely eradicate putrefaction were rewarded "with greater constancy than ever before," making surgeries possible that, otherwise, "would be simply homicidal." He was fearful that others might infer from Wood's lecture that he had lost faith in his own system by his relative silence during the two years since the Plymouth congress. Casting aspersions on Wood's ability, Lister set forth "that, of the many strangers who have witnessed my practice since his address was given, not one appears to have had any hesitation in arriving at the true explanation."[45]

How many visitors Lister entertained in a month is not known, but at least one of them resented his "sweeping assertion and insinuation." George Thomson, a surgeon in Oldham, depicted Lister as one who was unwilling to consider "the bare possibility of any failure," demanded blind acceptance of his results, was dogmatic, and could not be trusted because complications were "explained away." Disappointed, he

[43] Ibid., pp. 183–84, 185; W. J. Bishop, *The Early History of Surgery* (New York: Barnes & Noble, Inc., 1960), pp. 169–70.
[44] Joseph Lister to Robert Davidson Murray, 8 March 1877, Lister Papers, Library, Royal College of Surgeons of England, London, Drawer 5.
[45] Joseph Lister, "Professor Lister on Antiseptic Surgery," *The Lancet* (6 September 1873): 353–54.

left Edinburgh for conscience's sake, "with the last remnant of . . . belief in Professor Lister dissipated to the winds."[46] The physician who answered Thomson's allegations was J. Knowsley Thornton, one of Lister's former house-surgeons. Lister did not respond to Thomson and later explained his silence by saying that he was too busy trying to perfect his technique, but the attention he was getting from places other than London was also a factor. Thornton worked in London, but while studying under Lister, he had talked with Continental and American practitioners, who traveled to Scotland's capital, and learned that "an adverse opinion was a rare exception."[47]

Conspicuously missing from Thornton's list of areas represented by pilgrims to Edinburgh was England. No matter how much notoriety Lister got elsewhere, he would not feel vindicated without winning over his home country and especially the city of his birth. London, however, was to prove to be the most difficult bastion to take. The records from two of that city's hospitals in 1873 illustrate the peculiar problems encountered by metropolitan institutions and the uphill struggle Lister faced. At Guy's Hospital, for example, there were too many patients for surgeons to take the time required to properly implement the antiseptic method. Thus, the responsibility was delegated to dressers who also were hurried and, more importantly, might not "take a great interest in improvements."[48] The difficulty in St. Bartholomew's Hospital was that carbolic acid was simply used to wash wounds and as part of an oiled-lint dressing. Recovery was supposedly ensured "by extreme care and gentleness in the manipulation of the parts, by strict maintenance of rest, and by giving free exit to all serous discharge or matter."[49]

Lister's work was clearly cut out for him, and if he wanted to conquer the land to the south, he had to provide consistent, aggressive leadership. Ironically, Wood's speech elicited a commitment from Lister to bring forth, "in due time," more refinements in his system "together with evidence of their value in practice."[50] He undoubtedly knew that London stood as the last stronghold of opposition to him, and that prominent members of the medical community there, and elsewhere, were poised and ready to scrutinize every utterance from Edinburgh.

---

[46] George Thomson, "Antiseptic Surgery," *The Lancet* (20 September 1873): 432.
[47] J. Knowsley Thornton, "Antiseptic Surgery," *The Lancet* (27 September 1873): 470–71.
[48] J. Cooper Forster, "Clinical Records," *Guy's Hospital Reports,* Third Series, 18 (1873): 100–101.
[49] George W. Callender, "Two Years of Hospital Practice," *St. Bartholomew's Hospital Reports,* 9 (1873): 19.
[50] Lister, "Professor Lister," p. 353.

5. THEORETICAL ORIENTATION AS A FACTOR IN THE DIFFUSION OF LISTERISM

IN 1870 LISTER HAD GIVEN three reasons why English surgeons refused to imitate his system. Some practitioners summarily dismissed it because they equated it with the use of the caustic agent used to achieve it, others were careless in following the detailed practices required of his technique, and few surgeons wholeheartedly accepted the germ theory. The third factor was the most troublesome because the controversy over the germ theory remained unresolved during the entire time that Lister was gaining acceptance. Lister met the first objection by employing ever weaker solutions of carbolic acid and by using other antiseptic materials that were not so caustic. The second objection ceased to be a problem after Lister moved to London, where he could personally demonstrate his refined methods to the metropolitan medical establishment. Only in regard to the belief that living microscopic organisms caused disease was there relentless debate throughout Lister's career.

The first experimenter in the United Kingdom to enter the public arena on the question of airborne microorganisms, following Lister's announcement that the germ theory was the basis for his procedure, was John Hughes Bennett. Bennett was the senior professor of clinical medicine at the University of Edinburgh, and in an article for the *Edinburgh Medical Journal* entitled "The Atmospheric Germ Theory," he sided with Pasteur's most ardent opponent, F. A. Pouchet. Pouchet was a professor of natural history at Rouen and the author of a book on heterogenesis, or spontaneous generation of microorganisms; the broader term that was used for anything generated spontaneously was abiogenesis.[1] Bennett explained the appearance of microorganisms in rotting substances in terms of the molecular degeneration of those materials. His molecular theory of organization presumed an ongoing transformation of old tissues into new ones by both the aggregative and disintegrative action of molecules. Thus, Bennett taught that molecules became the building blocks of whole tissues, instead of cells, and that microorganisms could be spontaneously generated from the enlargement and combination of molecules.[2]

To Bennett the difference in formative molecules and those that constantly break down tissues was one of function, not structure, and he believed that diseases develop in the same way that tissues do.[3] In his judgment, diseases resulted from the physical properties of the air such as its chemical composition, density, and temperature. Bennett's physico-chemical views led him to reject Pasteur's argument that fermentation

---

[1] Heterogenesis was distinguished from homogenesis, which defined the vitality of microorganisms in terms of a parental source; those who held that sporules descended from pre-existing life were known as panspermatists, and they attributed fermentation and putrefaction to living matter, not chemical processes. John Hughes Bennett, "The Atmospheric Germ Theory," *Edinburgh Medical Journal* 13 (March 1868): 810, 812.

[2] Ibid., p. 831; J. K. Crellin, "The Dawn of the Germ Theory: Particles, Infection and Biology," in *Medicine and Science in the 1860s,* ed. F. N. L. Poynter (London: Wellcome Institute for the History of Medicine, 1968), pp. 59, 70.

[3] Bennett used the term histogenetic for those molecules that are constructive and histolytic for those that are destructive. John Harley Warner, "Therapeutic Explanation and the Edinburgh Bloodletting Controversy: Two Perspectives on the Medical Meaning of Science in the Mid-Nineteenth Century," *Medical History* 24 (July 1980): 248–50.

and putrefaction were caused by living organisms that the latter had isolated. Bennett briefly described Pasteur's experiment, which had produced the organisms, as one that was carried out

> by causing a current of air to pass through a glass tube in which a pledget of gun-cotton had been placed. This was then dissolved in ether, and the sediment allowed to collect in a watch-glass. This sediment, after being repeatedly washed, and allowed to remain in distilled water for twenty-four hours, is allowed to dry. A portion of the dried matter is then put upon a slide moistened with a weak solution of potash, and, being covered with another glass, is examined with the microscope.[4]

According to Bennett, Pasteur's method for securing the germs changed the very nature of the air, so that what was captured could not be conclusively identified as organic. The components of the dust acquired had also been found in minerals and, in Bennett's opinion, might be corpuscles of starch, clothing debris, by-products of combustion, vegetable or insect fragments, minuscule seeds, or animals that could only be detected with a microscope.[5]

Most of all, though, Bennett disagreed with Pasteur on the issue of temperature. The French chemist said that all microorganisms died at thirty degrees above the boiling point, but Pouchet demonstrated that they occurred on infusions which had been heated twenty degrees higher and that "animalcules and fungi" still formed at a temperature of two-hundred degrees centigrade. Pasteur also argued that extreme cold killed germs, which he showed by first boiling infusions and then subjecting them to a temperature of twenty-five to thirty degrees centigrade at high altitudes. Fifteen of twenty flasks he had prepared for this experiment remained free of microorganisms. Pouchet tried the same test with eight flasks at a higher altitude, and all of them became contaminated. When Pasteur complained that certain of his precautions had not been followed, such as not shaking the contents of the flasks and opening them with an instrument that had been heated, two of Pouchet's associates carefully repeated the experiment. Again, without exception, every flask exhibited contamination. According to Bennett, "so ended this part of the controversy."[6]

Bennett did not seem to realize that it was not just Pasteur's ability to isolate germs, but his success in keeping them from reappearing that proved his theory. Pasteur had asked the Academy of Sciences to verify this point during his dispute with Pouchet, but when the academy convened to observe demonstrations by both men, only Pasteur appeared. He successfully sterilized an infusion of yeast by boiling it to kill existing microbes and by preventing the access of dust from the air with a flask that had a curved neck. The arbitrators were, consequently, persuaded of the truth of Pasteur's theory. However, some cultures still could not be completely rid of microorganisms because a high enough temperature could not be applied to them. This was especially true of

---

[4] Bennett, "Germ Theory," pp. 818, 827.
[5] Ibid., p. 819.
[6] Ibid., pp. 827–28; Rene Vallery-Radot, *The Life of Pasteur* (Garden City, New York: Doubleday, Page & Company, 1926), pp. 95–99, 104–106.

infusions of hay. Pouchet could have used such infusions to support his position, since living organisms would have reappeared even after the infusions were subjected to an amount of heat thought to be incompatible with existence. Had he done so, it would have seemed that living matter was being spontaneously generated.[7]

Bennett did seize on the inability of heat to sterilize hay cultures and showed that boiling them did not prevent them from becoming cloudy and forming fungi. He also criticized all of Pasteur's experiments from the previous eight years as "contradictory and ingenious," specifically challenging those with yeast. Pasteur had shown that both fresh yeast and the ashes of yeast were susceptible to fermentation when exposed to the atmosphere. The reason this was considered contradictory by Bennett was because he thought Pasteur meant that the yeasts were the sources of fermentation, even though the Frenchman had repeatedly said that the cause of fermentation was living microbes. Also, since Pouchet and his two associates had produced contamination at temperatures well above those compatible with life, Bennett concluded that ferments and the causes of putrefaction must be non-living matter. Moreover, he thought that Pasteur had proved the same point by causing fermentation with the ashes of yeast, which were obviously dead.[8]

If Bennett considered Pasteur's findings to be inconsistent, Lister certainly did not. As a matter of fact, Lister's introductory lecture at Edinburgh on November 8, 1869, was on the germ theory, and throughout his tenure there he called Pasteur his master. His speech was given in a classroom that had been used for chemistry, appropriate since it was a professor of chemistry in Glasgow who had initially acquainted Lister with the writings of Pasteur.[9] The oration was probably intended as a rebuttal to Bennett, and Lister discussed how putrefaction was caused by "living organisms developed from germs floating in the atmosphere as constituents of its dust." He elaborated on the origin of those organisms, saying that they came from "pre-existing similar organisms." Using the broadest meaning of the word "germs," that which germinates, Lister looked upon "micro- organisms as very plastic and tentatively proposed that septic organisms were the buds of yeast."[10]

To whatever extent Lister's decision to concentrate on the germ theory in his address was predicated on Bennett's rejection of it, his comments were also based on his opponents having turned their attention away from the antiseptic technique. They now focused on Pasteur's theory, "the central dogma of antisepsis."[11] Bennett definitely considered Lister's remarks to be a challenge to what he had been teaching and asked him, "Where are these little beasts? Show them to us, and we shall believe in them. Has anyone seen them yet?"[12] Bennett was a microscopist but apparently only saw what he wanted to see. Lister refused to respond to him, and one historian implies that it was because he considered Bennett's questions to be absurd.[13]

---

[7] D. Berry Hart, "An Address on Pasteur and Lister," *The British Medical Journal* (13 December 1902): 1839.
[8] Bennett, "Germ Theory," pp. 824–25, 828–29.
[9] John Chiene, "Edinburgh Royal Infirmary, 1869–1877," *The British Medical Journal* (13 December 1902): 1848.
[10] Christopher Lawrence and Richard Dixey, "Practising on Principle: Joseph Lister and the Germ Theories of Disease," in *Medical Theory, Surgical Practice,* ed. Christopher Lawrence (London: Routledge, 1992), pp. 173, 210; Joseph Lister, *The Collected Papers of Joseph, Baron Lister,* 2 vols. (Oxford: The Clarendon Press, 1909), 2:479, 482.
[11] Richard B. Fisher, *Joseph Lister, 1827–1912* (New York: Stein and Day, 1977), pp. 121, 134, 179.
[12] Quoted in Knut Haeger, *The Illustrated History of Surgery* (New York: Bell Publishing Company, 1988), p. 211.
[13] Ibid; Warner, "Therapeutic Explanation," p. 241.

The most prominent man in the United Kingdom willing to invest his time in arguing with those who did not believe in the existence of living germs was John Tyndall, Professor of Natural Philosophy at the Royal Institution in London. Thomas Huxley, president of the British Association for the Advancement of Science and the leading proponent of Darwinism, was better known and devoted his presidential address to the controversy in 1870, but he was not able to give his undivided attention to it. He did support the germ theory and even coined the term biogenesis to mean that all life comes from previous life, but he also "cautioned that microorganisms possess variable heat resistance and that such resistance is influenced by physical and chemical characteristics of the culture medium."[14]

Unlike Huxley, Tyndall could make the long-term commitment to experimentation which was ultimately necessary to resolve whether or not life originated from non-living sources. He looked upon H. Charlton Bastian, an early physician of neurology who practiced at the National Hospital of the Epileptic and Paralysed, as his leading antagonist. Bastian was also a physician and professor of pathological anatomy at University College Hospital, Lister's alma mater. He initiated a debate with Tyndall in April, 1870, through a letter-writing campaign to *The Times.* Tyndall later labeled the ensuing exchange a "paper war." Tyndall had incited Bastian by opening the new year with a highly publicized lecture entitled "On Dust and Disease."[15] (See Figure 9.)

In his lecture, Tyndall stated that the dust of the air was organic and combustible. He defined dust as any particles that were visible in a beam of sunlight and observed that they could not be seen in air passed over an open flame because they were extinguished. He went on to say, "If the air were sent too rapidly through the flame, a fine blue cloud was noticed. This was the smoke of the organic particles." Furthermore, Tyndall emphasized the overwhelming number of particles in the air and described them as "churning . . . in our lungs every hour and minute of our lives." He expressed amazement that so few of them apparently caused death but then referred to the contagious ones that obviously covered surgical instruments, since heat was not applied to destroy them. He concluded by agreeing with the findings of Pasteur, Lister, and William Budd, the physician from Bristol who proved that typhoid was caused by a specific organism, and recommended that "cotton-wool respirators" be used to keep germs from being breathed.[16]

The lecture was so controversial, the editor of *The Lancet* wrote that Tyndall had "disturbed the mind of the general public by his sensational endeavour to ventilate . . . a question that is still amongst the most uncertain of those by which men of science are perplexed."[17] The question James G. Wakley was alluding to was the debate over the germ theory, but he attacked Tyndall's method for trying to prove it, saying that "the less we have of it in medicine and surgery the better for ourselves and the public." Wakley simply noted that the cilia of the respiratory system were better filters of the air's impurities than cotton-wool. Concerning germs, he wrote that "no such

[14] Glenn Vandervliet, *Microbiology and the Spontaneous Generation Debate During the 1870's* (Lawrence, Kansas: Coronado Press, 1971), pp. 13–14, 36.
[15] Ibid., pp. 23–24, 54; J. K. Crellin, "The Problem of Heat Resistance of Micro-Organisms in the British Spontaneous Generation Controversies of 1860–1880," *Medical History* 10 (January 1966): 50, 52, 56–57.
[16] Jonathan Hutchinson, "Dust and Disease," *The British Medical Journal* (29 January 1870): 118–19.
[17] James G. Wakley, "Germs," *The Lancet* (14 May 1870): 704.

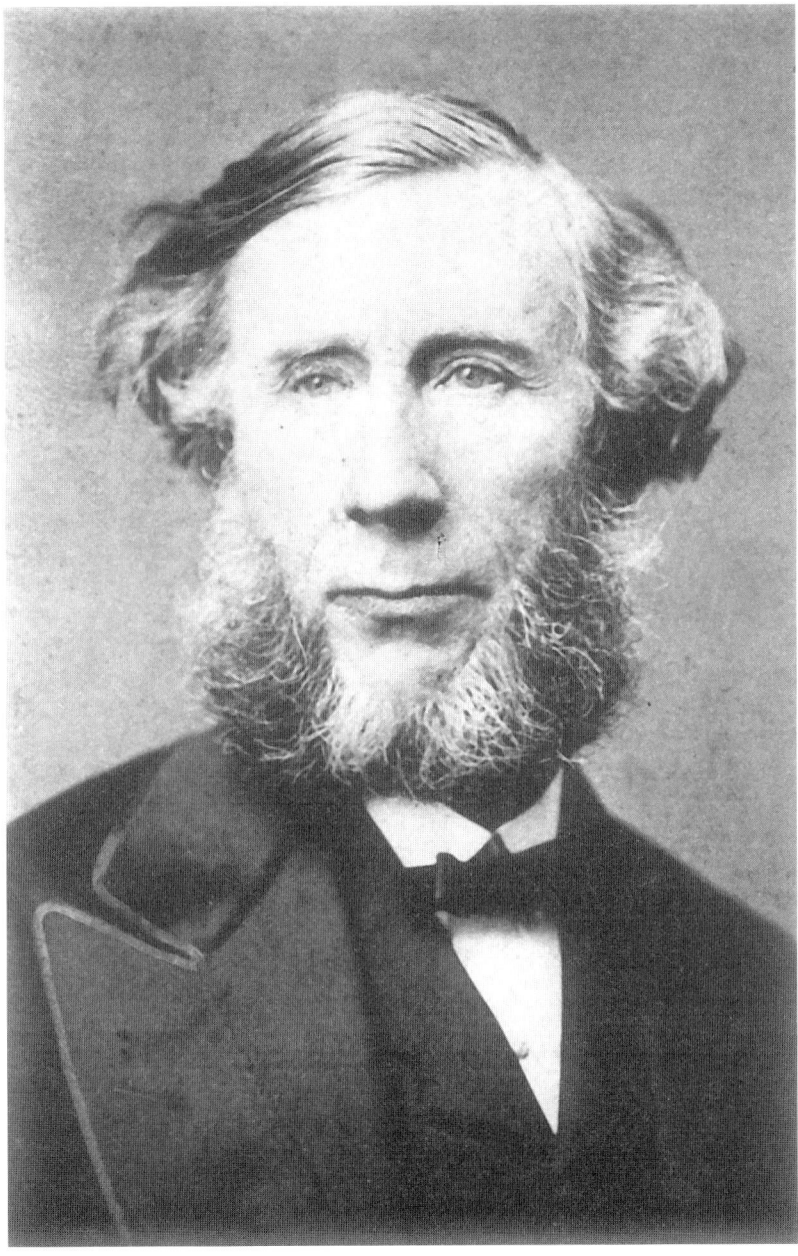

Figure 9. John Tyndall

things have as yet been seen—that to the naturalist, they are as purely imaginary as the sea serpent." Because Tyndall was a natural philosopher Wakley concluded that he had spoken "on a subject of which he can know next to nothing."[18] However, Wakley looked upon Bastian differently. Of the pathologist he penned, "His strength as against Professor Tyndall lies in his mastery of the subject, and in his power to avoid errors into which the eminent physicist has unconsciously fallen."[19]

Based on what he had learned, though, Tyndall later suggested that surgeons use heated instruments to lance abscesses. Wakley considered such advice, founded on a belief in the germ theory, to be ridiculous but added that he no longer thought that spontaneous generation and the germ theory "were antagonistic and incompatible." Indeed, he speculated that there was a "very high probability that both these views will at no distant time be established." He thought that if either theory "were true exclusively, the evidence of its truth would not be difficult to obtain." Because of the great discrepancies in them, therefore, he was convinced that parts of both would be accepted philosophically. Also, Wakley now held both Bastian and Tyndall at arm's length. He stated that Bastian's experiments, especially those involving saline solutions in which living organisms appeared after air was expelled and heat was administered, were "open to the obvious objection that they may have been in some way erroneously conducted."[20]

Whether or not Bastian's tests were performed properly, all honest searchers for truth recognized the need for additional experimentation to resolve the controversy over spontaneous generation and the germ theory. Wakley assented to the necessity for more research, but was so biased in his own opinion that he prejudiced his readers against the possibility of ever controlling disease-causing agents. He showed his unscientific attitude in the matter when he pessimistically declared that:

> It is certain that the air around us, especially the air of populous places, contains much floating matter of a noxious character, many floating germs of common fungi, possibly many germs productive of special forms of disease. It is certain that the mechanical exclusion of such impurities, or their destruction by chemical agents, will often be highly advantageous. It is also certain that we cannot exclude in this way all the noxious agents that produce animalcular life or zymotic disease; and we shall, in the present state of knowledge, only waste time and lose labour if we aim at the unattainable by an accumulation of minute precautions.[21]

Those who believed in spontaneous generation looked upon attempts to refute their explanation for the origin of life as exercises in futility, confident that their doctrine was theoretically unassailable. Their unwillingness to subject their convictions to repeated scientific scrutiny contributed to the acceptance of the germ theory because they spent their time philosophizing and pontificating while inquisitive researchers produced undeniable, replicable evidence that supported Pasteur's findings.

---

[18] James G. Wakley, "Professor Tyndall as a Pathologist," *The Lancet* (16 April 1870): 555–56.
[19] James G. Wakley, "Professor Tyndall," *The Lancet* (30 April 1870): 626.
[20] Wakley, "Germs," pp. 704–05.
[21] Ibid.

Benjamin Ward Richardson, a physician at St. John's Hospital for Skin Diseases in London, was an extreme example of a physician who despised experimenters. Instead of testing theories to arrive at preventive measures for disease, "he relied on the combined effects of sanitation and salvation, on outer and inner cleansing."[22] The two were one and the same thing to Richardson, and pain served the purpose of alerting its recipient to stop making either hygienic or ethical mistakes. He said it was fruitless to "try to master pain by entering into experimental conflict with Nature on her own ground," and he castigated "all elaborate experiments for the prevention of disease" because they were "mysterious additions to evil which ought not to exist."[23] To his credit, though, it should be stressed that much of his life was spent in trying to abrogate pain; he not only invented a "lethal chamber for the painless killing of dogs and cats" but also introduced a number of anesthetics to relieve their suffering. An accurate description of Richardson's views on medicine, especially vaccinations, has been provided by one writer's contrast of the methods of sanitarians like Edwin Chadwick and those of researchers like Pasteur:

> Preventive medicine of the Chadwick pattern got rid of "impurity" and "pollution"—words much used in the pulpit and burdened with complex meanings in ordinary speech; but the preventive medicine of Jenner and Pasteur actually introduced "impurity" into the body, or worse still, into the blood, a fluid of mystic significance and the peculiar vehicle of life. With the special sexual connotation of the word, "morals," the charge was complete. A healthy life was a "clean" life.[24]

On October 31, 1870, the Medical Society of London discussed a paper Richardson had written, entitled "On the Medical Aspects of the Germ Theory." In it he said nothing about the origin of life, but called Pasteur's theory "untenable." He believed in a "physical doctrine of organic poisons . . . capable of being introduced into the body from without, or of being generated in its own secretions." The poisons were "dead organic matter" that could be transmitted as solids or in water and air.[25] Richardson's ideas became known as the glandular theory, and he believed that the "organic poisons" were chemical in nature. He claimed to have isolated one such poisonous particle, which he named a "septine." He also considered the source of all secretions to be albumin, a product of blood. He looked upon himself as a modifier of the ideas of John Snow, the surgeon from London who proved that cholera was caused by a specific organism. Snow had referred to the organism as a "cholera cell" and maintained that it came from cells that already existed. By the time Richardson wrote his paper on the germ theory, the topic of interest among cell theorists was not the cell itself, but protoplasm, the living matter of the cell. Richardson fully expounded his

[22] M. Jeanne Peterson, *The Medical Profession in Mid-Victorian London* (Berkeley: University of California Press, 1978), p. 265; Lloyd G. Stevenson, "Science down the Drain: On the Hostility of Certain Sanitarians to Animal Experimentation, Bacteriology and Immunology," *Bulletin of the History of Medicine* 29 (January–February 1955): 8–9.
[23] Quoted in Stevenson, "Science down the Drain," p. 13.
[24] Ibid., pp. 7, 14.
[25] James G. Wakley, "Medical Society of London," *The Lancet* (29 October 1870): 606–607.

views on communicable diseases in his *Diseases of Modern Life,* which was published six years after his paper on the medical aspects of the germ theory.[26]

Richardson's argument against the germ theory was summed up by Wakley, who reported that "the hypothetical germs being omnipresent, reproductive, and indestructible by conditions that are fatal to higher organisms . . . would supplant all others, and that the life of the universe would come to consist of germs alone." Richardson then had the audacity to point out that when the germ theory was taken to its logical conclusion, "it undergoes a *reductio ad absurdum.*"[27] Clearly, it was Richardson's views that were ridiculous, and they became even more ludicrous as he responded to the members of the London Medical Society who discussed his paper. He prophesied that those who supported the germ theory would soon cast it aside, like those who discard items on a manure heap, and would agree among themselves to keep their mouths shut about it. He could not, however, keep silent on the use of carbolic acid, claiming that the success of those who did not employ it was as great as those who did. He said no proof existed that fermentation occurred in diseases.[28]

Suffice it to say, the followers of Pasteur and Lister in Great Britain were not content to remain quiet either. A. E. Sansom, who wrote the first book on the antiseptic system, was particularly vocal in opposing critics who believed in spontaneous generation. He rejected the ideas of Richardson entirely and defended the "diffusion of a volatile antiseptic in air" to destroy "disease-germs." This was an obvious reference to the carbolic-acid spray, which Lister did not mention in writing until December 31, 1870; ironically, the first sprayer Lister used was a modified version of one that had been invented by Richardson. Sansom was criticized by an anonymous opponent of the germ theory for basing his assertions on microscopical evidence gleaned from examining putrid discharges of wounds instead of diseases themselves. The critic admonished him to test contagious and infectious diseases and told him that disease-causing agents could only be immobilized by subjecting them to a temperature of four-hundred degrees or more. Also, Sansom's detractor viewed acceptance of the germ theory as precluding pathological examinations, especially of "morbid blood products . . . leaving for research only the fungi and animalcules which grow in the barren external highways."[29]

Interestingly, research into "fungi" had originated the concept of germs as causes of disease in the United Kingdom. In one of his editorials Wakley attributed that idea to Budd. Budd had written a letter to *The Times* in 1849, suggesting that cholera was caused by a distinct species of living organisms that appeared to be fungoid in nature. He further intimated that if these "cholera fungi" were real, "their germs or spores might be the means of propagating infection." Accepting the notion of spores, Wakley

---

[26] Crellin, "Dawn of the Germ Theory," pp. 62–63; Benjamin Ward Richardson, *Diseases of Modern Life* (New York: D. Appleton and Company, 1876), pp. 88–89, 94–95.

[27] James G. Wakley, "Germs in George-Street," *The Lancet* (5 November 1870): 643–44.

[28] Ibid; Ernest Hart, "Medical Society of London," *The British Medical Journal* (19 November 1870): 566–67.

[29] Hart, "Medical Society," pp. 566–67; Fisher, *Joseph Lister,* p. 184; quoted in Forward Progress [pseud.], "Backward Progress: The Germ Theory," *The Lancet* (20 January 1872): 99; Richardson used a sprayer to administer "a finely atomized cloud of sulphuric ether on to the patient's skin, where it immediately vaporized, and in so doing refrigerated the superficial tissues sufficiently for all sorts of surgical operations to be done." Arthur Salusbury MacNalty, *A Biography of Sir Benjamin Ward Richardson* (London: Harvey & Blythe, Ltd., 1950), p. 42.

dogmatically proclaimed that "it has become manifest to most thinking people that a belief in germs, by which we mean ovular germs, as the cause of spreading diseases, involves the absolutely unreserved acceptance of the doctrine of spontaneous generation." He based his proclamation on apparently "complete and irrefragable" evidence that spreading "diseases may originate in places to which they cannot have been brought."[30]

Though Wakley did not enthusiastically encourage experimentation, calling researches that attempted to rid the atmosphere of disease-causing agents a waste of time, he did endeavor to define terminology and called upon those who supported the germ theory to "discard the use of words of doubtful meaning." He directed the attention of his readers to the observations of John Burdon-Sanderson, with which he said he was able to "fully coincide." Burdon-Sanderson, a professor of practical physiology at University College, the same school where Bastian taught, had voiced his "general assent" to Richardson's paper.[31] He also agreed with the findings of Bastian, especially those revealed in the latter's book, *The Beginnings of Life: Being Some Account of the Nature, Modes of Origin and Transformations of Lower Organisms.*

Bastian's book, published in 1872, recorded an experiment in which urine was heated to one-hundred and ten degrees centigrade, ten degrees higher than water's boiling point. The acidity of the urine was then neutralized. Nevertheless, it later clouded, indicating the presence of living organisms. Bastian was sure that he had disproved the atmospheric germ theory. In actuality, he used water that had been distilled to dissolve potash, the substance which was put into the urine to neutralize it. The water may have had some hidden bacteria in it, and there are dormant bacteria in urine which can survive temperatures of more than one-hundred and sixty degrees centigrade. Regardless of these shortcomings in his arguments, Bastian's experiment did significantly bolster the case for spontaneous generation and "indirectly cast doubt on Lister's ability to exclude germs by his antiseptic method."[32]

One year after the appearance of Bastian's monograph, Burdon-Sanderson wrote an article of his own on the origin of bacteria. The experiments on which it was based were essentially the same as those performed by John Hughes Bennett five years earlier. Infusions containing vegetable or animal substance were placed in hermetically sealed flasks and heated above the boiling point. Since some living organisms continued to survive under such conditions, Burdon-Sanderson concluded that germ theorists were wrong on two counts. They were mistaken when they said that boiling destroyed the vitality of bacteria and when they asserted that fungi do not move through the atmosphere. If flasks prepared in this manner still showed active organisms after the infusions had been boiled, then Burdon-Sanderson assumed that the water conveyed the bacteria. This would indicate that what was in the air outside was something other than bacteria, namely fungi. Using Wakley's definition of germs, he ended his article with a rhetorical challenge to believers in the germ theory:

---

[30] Margaret Pelling, *Cholera, Fever and English Medicine, 1825–1865* (Oxford: Oxford University Press, 1978), p. 170; Wakley, "Germs," (19 November 1870): 714.
[31] Wakley, "Germs," (19 November 1870): 714; Wakley, "George-Street," p. 644.
[32] H. Charlton Bastian, *The Beginnings of Life: Being Some Account of the Nature, Modes of Origin and Transformations of Lower Organisms,* 2 vols. (New York: D. Appleton and Co., 1872), 1:344–99; Fisher, *Joseph Lister,* pp. 181–82.

Are you now, therefore, going to say that the temperature of boiling water is probably insufficient to devitalise the parents of bacteria? or do you feel inclined to think that, after all, it may be true that bacteria can arise without the pre-existence of germs in the ordinary sense of this term?[33]

Burdon-Sanderson was so highly respected that when Lister decided to join this philosophical wrangling over the germ theory he dealt mainly with Burdon-Sanderson's ideas, not those of Bennett or Bastian. (See Figure 10.)

Lister systematically defended the germ theory in a speech that he delivered to the Royal Society of Edinburgh on April 7, 1873; an expanded version of it was finally published two years later. It shows that he had a clear understanding of Pasteur's theories as well as those of Pasteur's opponents. Lister began his argument by stating that "organic substances, when left exposed under ordinary circumstances, undergo alterations in their qualities." His explanation for this phenomenon followed. "The Germ Theory," he proclaimed,

supposes that the organisms are the causes of the changes; that the germs of these minute living things, diffusible in proportion to their minuteness, are omnipresent in the world around us, and are sure to gain access to any exposed organic substance; and, having thus reached it, develop if it prove a favourable *nidus,* and by their growth determine the chemical changes; and further, that these organisms, minute though they appear to us, form no exception to the general law of living beings, that they originate from similar beings by parentage.[34]

He then listed three alternative explanations for those changes: the influence of oxygen on organic substances; the action of chemical ferments on them, "the organisms being regarded as accidental accompaniments"; and the possibility of inorganic substances producing causative agents through spontaneous generation, "admitting perhaps the fermentative agency of the organisms."

Turning his attention to more immediate concerns, Lister acknowledged that Burdon-Sanderson's results, which appeared to show that bacteria are conveyed by water but not air, would have far-reaching consequences on the way he practiced surgery, if they proved to be "strictly correct." He described the details of Burdon-Sanderson's experiments as "striking" but expressed his disbelief in their exactness and confessed that he found them "too good to be true." By these remarks, he meant that he could forego the use of the carbolic-acid spray, if indeed, bacteria are not conveyed by air. Lister admitted that being able to do so would bring him great joy. Relying on urine as his medium, like Bastian, he performed experiments of his own to expose Burdon-Sanderson's errors.

Lister did not initially boil the urine to remove contamination. Instead, he prepared the skin around the opening of a patient's urethra antiseptically and collected the fluid waste as it was voided. Lister placed the urine in six wine glasses that had

---

[33] John Burdon-Sanderson, "The Origin of Bacteria," *The British Medical Journal* (1 February 1873): 120–21.
[34] Lister, *Collected Papers,* 1:275–76.

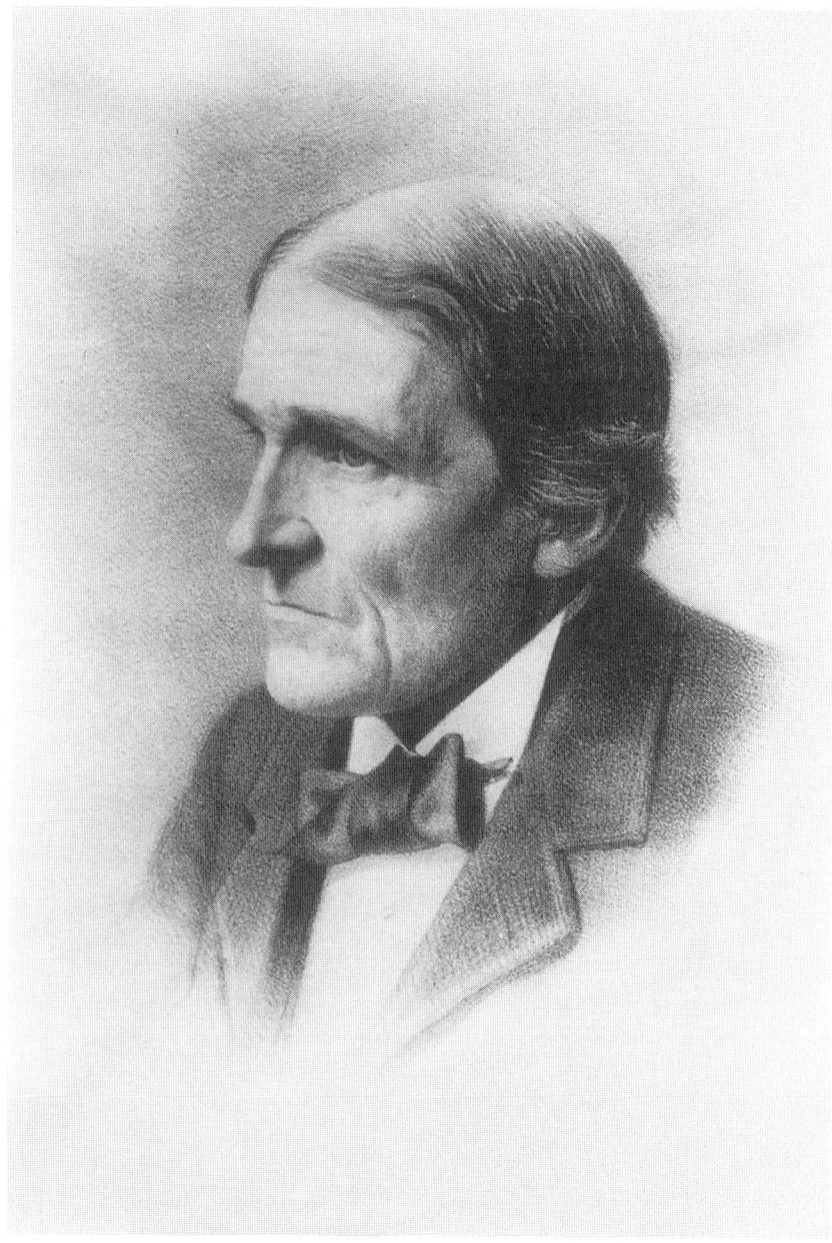

Figure 10. John Burdon-Sanderson

been heated to a temperature in excess of one-hundred degrees centigrade and then cooled. Various amounts of water were added to three of them, two of which were covered. Two additional glasses were also covered with a glass plate that had been heated like the wine glasses, but no water was added to them. The last of the six was left open and free of water.

After two days, the period which Burdon-Sanderson allowed for his tests, the first three glasses all showed evidence of bacteria, but the three which had no water in them did not. These results were identical to those of Burdon-Sanderson. Lister, though, waited an additional twelve hours and bacteria formed on the water-free glass that had been left open. Also, after a third day, he uncovered the other two glasses that were free of water and one of them rendered bacterial growth "in the course of a few days." He was persuaded that if he had been more meticulous in his method, he could have kept bacteria from forming at all in those glasses that were covered and water-free. Thus, Lister was convinced that bacteria were indeed air-borne and that "the healthy living tissues" of a patient could prevent them from having a deleterious effect.[35]

Six months after speaking to the Royal Society of Edinburgh, another presentation of Lister's, entitled "A Further Contribution to the Natural History of Bacteria and the Germ Theory of Fermentative Changes," was immediately published in the *Quarterly Journal of Microscopical Science.* By then he was much surer of his conclusions because of his replication of them and emphatically maintained that "any classification of bacteria hitherto made . . . based upon absolute morphological characters, is entirely untrustworthy."[36] In other words, germs could not be identified and categorized on the basis of their form or shape alone. This was the same thing that Bennett had said about molecules. Their action, or lack thereof, had to be taken into consideration also.[37]

It has been suggested by two revisionists that rather than defending Pasteur's germ theory, Lister was proposing another "full-blown germ theory of putrefaction," which he used "as an explanation of *all* contagious diseases." They stress that it "was *not* a theory of specific organisms causing specific diseases, quite the reverse. Contagious diseases were highly variable because of the great environmentally determined plasticity of organisms." These interpreters base their analysis on the tendency, according to Lister, of non-virulent microorganisms to develop into detrimental ones by contacting the putrefying discharges of wounds.[38]

Yet, because Lister did not have a twentieth-century understanding of microbiology does not mean that his thinking was essentially different from Pasteur's. He was concerned with the specificity of microorganisms once they were no longer benign. When Pasteur personally applied his theory to medicine five years later, he made statements very similar to Lister's. Tracing the development of a "vibrion of septicemia" from an innocuous microorganism to a latent, "corpuscular" germ to a virulent bacteria, Pasteur concluded that "due to extraneous conditions, organisms can change considerably their form and properties."[39]

Upon Lister's insistence, Wakley examined his findings and surmised that he had not disproved the theory of spontaneous generation at all! In fact, Wakley argued that Lister's experiments were not relevant to the debate over the origin of disease-causing

[35] Ibid., 1:276–79.
[36] Ibid., 1:309–10.
[37] James G. Wakley, "Professor Lister and the Germ Theory," *The Lancet* (11 October 1873): 530.
[38] Lawrence and Dixey, "Practising on principle," pp. 178–79; Lister, *Collected Papers,* 1:304, 333.
[39] Karel B. Absolon, Mary J. Absolon, and Ralph Zientek, "From Antisepsis to Asepsis: Louis Pasteur's publication on 'The Germ Theory and Its Application to Medicine and Surgery,'" *Review of Surgery* 27 (July–August 1970): 248–50, 253.

microorganisms. He also questioned Lister's wisdom in leaving the discussion of his technique to engage in the germ theory controversy. He knew that defending both his technique and the doctrine on which it was based put Lister in double jeopardy and left him with only two choices. Either he had to refute both Bastian and Burdon-Sanderson, "or else he must change the theoretical basis upon which his system has hitherto reposed, and must allow it to rest upon the broader physical theory, rather than upon the narrow and exclusive vital theory of fermentation." The theory Wakley considered to be more general was the one that explained changes in organisms as chemical processes when they led to disease.[40]

After he was presented with this argument, Lister retreated somewhat and said that his primary intention had been to illuminate the "nature and habits" of organisms that cause fermentation. Wakley then hastened to point out that the particles Lister had discovered in his experiments could just as easily be "mere dead organic fragments rather than living germs of pre-existing organisms."[41] By 1874 much confusion existed among microscopists because of experiments which seemed to indicate that boiling would not guarantee the sterilization of all media. Non-acidic solutions were hard to sterilize, and experiments performed on these solutions "fostered the concept of the possibility of heat resistant organisms and hence must have created a favourable climate for the recognition of the role of resistant spores." However, the existence of such organisms had no place in the germ theory of that day.[42]

Even more uncertainty was caused by efforts to understand the taxonomy of bacteria. If Darwin could devise a system for classifying plants and animals, why was it so difficult to group bacteria? Were they vegetative or were they from the animal kingdom? Tyndall subscribed to the latter grouping, but others looked upon all bacteria "as strictly forming part of the vegetable kingdom."[43] Those who subscribed to the vegetable theory of disease held that there were "different species or varieties of fungi corresponding to the several contagious maladies." They thought that disease germs were composed of germinal matter, and thus, "must necessarily be of a vegetable nature and have sprung from vegetable organisms, or have originated spontaneously."[44] Bastian, of course, did not concur with either classification, but maintained his position that bacteria were the results of the deterioration of tissues.[45]

Additional arguments against the germ theory stemmed from the fact that few diseases had been directly linked to microorganisms. Arguing that a leap of faith had taken Pasteur's followers from the conclusion that germs were the cause of fermentation to the assumption that all contagious diseases originated with microscopic organisms, Bastian singled out Lister and indicated that all of the conflicting opinions in the British Isles on the origin of bacteria were in opposition to the theory on which he had based his antiseptic technique. Fevers were especially troublesome for germ

---

[40] Wakley, "Professor Lister and the Germ Theory," pp. 529–30.

[41] Ibid., (25 October 1873): 600–601.

[42] In the 1860s and 1870s germs were generally construed to be the predecessors, regardless of their nature, of known microorganisms; they were looked upon as fragments in the atmosphere, either large enough to be isolated and studied with the assistance of a microscope or so minute that they were only discernible as interferences in lightbeams. Crellin, "Heat Resistance," pp. 50, 56.

[43] W. A. Hollis, "What is a Bacterium?," *The Lancet* (21 November 1874): 725.

[44] Lionel S. Beale, *Disease Germs; Their Nature and Origin,* 2d ed. (London: J. & A. Churchill, 1872), pp. 8–9.

[45] James G. Wakley, "The Debate on the Germ Theory of Disease," *The Lancet* (27 March 1875): 445.

theorists, and concerning the relationship of Pasteur's concept to them Bastian simply stated, "No positive facts of much weight seem to be forthcoming in favour of the germ theory as applied to contagious fevers." While many organisms could be found in putrefying tissues, Bastian agreed with Lionel S. Beale, who also said that bacteria derive from the decomposition of tissue but added "that all the tissues of man and higher animals are densely interpenetrated by undeveloped and indistinguishable germs of the lowest organisms." Beale was a microscopist at King's College in London and had written two books in 1870, respectively entitled *Disease Germs; their Supposed Nature* and *Disease Germs; their Real Nature.* Bastian believed that such germs were generated spontaneously from the decayed tissues and were not the result of biological reproduction.[46]

Specifically, Beale held that disease-causing germs were alive and that they were fragments of decomposed protoplasm, a semifluid substance considered to be the physical basis of life; it had the power to move spontaneously and to reproduce itself. He also determined that bacteria were atmospherically transmitted and that they caused diseases by entering the bloodstream. Beale's greatest contribution to the discussion of germs was the fact that he was the first to offer evidence that all diseases were associated with distinct microorganisms, even though he could not isolate those organisms from other living particles. He included drawings in his books of the fragments he had seen with his microscope.

It is likely that Beale's ideas motivated Burdon-Sanderson to conduct more detailed experiments, which he described in his 1870 introduction to a bluebook written by John Simon. At that time Simon was the medical officer for the Privy Council, which not only commissioned Burdon-Sanderson's research but also oversaw the licensing of medical practitioners. This particular government publication reported "results which, for the first time, seemed to prove that the particles were the infectious factors in disease." Burdon-Sanderson had successfully "separated, by diffusion, the particles in vaccine lymph." He then vaccinated two test groups of fifty-seven children each, one with ordinary lymph and the other with lymph minus the particles. Forty-seven of those who had received ordinary lymph tested positive, while only five of the other children experienced reactions. He described the particles as "mainly, but not exclusively composed of albuminous matter."[47]

Bastian was not easy to convince, however, and on April 6, 1875, he delivered a long address on the germ theory of disease to the Pathological Society of London in which he took issue with Beale and Burdon-Sanderson. From his vantage point they were both "germ theorists," and it is true that by that time the experiments conducted by Burdon-Sanderson had led him to believe in living particles as the cause of putrefaction. Burdon-Sanderson had even gone so far as to retract his earlier opinions on the subject and now alleged that bacteria were absorbed easily into the bloodstream "from the intestine by lymphatics" and "from without . . . through the bronchi and the lungs." However, he still argued that there were no germs in healthy blood because he believed that the presence of bacteria was clear evidence of outside contamination.

---

[46] H. Charlton Bastian, "The Discussion at the Pathological Society," *The Lancet* (20 March 1875): 410.

[47] Crellin, "Dawn of the Germ Theory," pp. 63–65; James G. Wakley, "Pathological Society of London," *The Lancet* (15 May 1875): 683.

Cleverly, before Bastian concluded his presentation, he labored to establish "common ground" with Burdon-Sanderson and Beale against Pasteur and Lister. Speaking for himself and his newly chosen associates, he said,

> We are agreed as to the fact that bacteria are abundantly present within the body, or that they may appear therein under certain conditions independent of any immediate external contamination—however much we may differ amongst ourselves as to the interpretation of their presence, actual or possible.[48]

Bastian stated that the main point of contention between him and Lister was the latter's refusal to admit that bacteria "naturally exist within the body." He then declared his suspicion that Pasteur would ultimately agree with him and concede "his long-postponed acceptance of doctrines of 'spontaneous generation.'"[49]

Although Bastian feigned camaraderie with Burdon-Sanderson, the relationship was one-sided, and when Burdon-Sanderson responded Bastian must have been shocked. Burdon-Sanderson showed just how far he had distanced himself from his previous ideas when he said, "It is impossible to suppose that the moment a patient became febrile these organisms were spontaneously generated, and that the moment he ceased to be febrile they were spontaneously annihilated."[50]

Wakley actually sided with Burdon-Sanderson and called Bastian's view a "preconceived theory." He compared Bastian to those who reject everything and then demand confirmation of what has been denied. Wakley also spoke satirically of Bastian, telling his readers that "it is unnecessary to follow him in his arguments as to the mode of origin of bacteria if they possess so little importance as he ascribes to them."[51] However, Bastian had his supporters too, and they included J. Dougall, one of Lister's former students and one of the leading advocates of the antiseptic method.

Dougall, a surgeon in Glasgow who voiced respect for Lister as a teacher whose theory had been "well drummed" into him, referred to Bastian's address as "apparently exhaustive." He surmised that it was persuasive enough to convert those who were undecided about the germ theory and to strengthen the faith of those who were opposed to it. If anything was apparent, though, it was his blind faith in Bastian because he parroted his words almost verbatim, saying that bacteria are already present in the body and that there are none in the air. J. Knowsley Thornton, one of Lister's former house-surgeons, was also impressed with Bastian's argument and for the most part agreed with it, writing that it had "shut out to a great extent the question." He parenthetically inserted his conviction that germs were not living organisms, but he did recognize them as "bacteria floating in the atmosphere."[52] These dissenting views by those closely associated with Lister tended to separate the debate over the germ theory from questions relating to the usefulness of the antiseptic technique.

---

[48] H. Charlton Bastian, "An Address on the Germ Theory of Disease; being a Discussion of the Relation of Bacteria and Allied Organisms to Virulent Inflammations and Specific Contagious Fevers," *The Lancet* (10 April 1875): 501, 504–505, 507.
[49] Ibid., pp. 507, 509.
[50] Wakley, "Pathological Society," (10 April 1875): 511, 513.
[51] Wakley, "Debate," (10 April 1875): 514.
[52] Wakley, "Pathological Society," (24 April 1875): 573, 575–76, 579.

Bastian was not content to spread his gospel only among the members of the medical profession. He attacked John Simon for printing Burdon-Sanderson's findings in a bluebook, accusing him of accepting the germ theory for all practical purposes. Simon concurred with Burdon-Sanderson that bacteria have a characteristic shape, are abundant, reproduce themselves, are "not congeneric with the animal body in which they are found," and as organic matter "are probably the essence or an inseparable part of the essence of all the contagia of disease." Bastian called upon him and others to be cognizant of "the facts of contagion" but "not to be pure contagionists."[53]

Wakley agreed with Bastian that Burdon-Sanderson was in sympathy with the germ theory, but he accused Burdon-Sanderson of being hesitant to defend it. Wakley also acknowledged the "one-sided character" of the presentations at the Pathological Society of London, specifically noting the absence of proponents of the germ theory such as Lister and Simon. He then ended his remarks on the state of the debate by reiterating his personal opinion of Pasteur's theory as well as his views on Lister's technique. He was fairly dogmatic, although a slight shift in his original thinking on the germ theory is discernible. He wrote that

> it must be confessed that the *de novo* origin of specific diseases is in many instances the only alternative, and more probable than the germ theory; but it can hardly be expected that the upholders of the latter theory will be inclined to go further than this at present, the evidence in favour of the cause and dissemination of contagious disease by means of specific germs being so strong as it is. Nor, indeed, whether the hypothesis of all-pervading germs or that of obscure and occult physico-chemical processes be the true one, it happily cannot affect the practical value of the use of antiseptics in surgery, or stay the progress of preventive medicine.[54]

This small crack in the armor of spontaneous generationism was about to become a gaping hole as incontrovertible facts supporting the germ theory began to assail it.

---

[53] Ibid., (15 May 1875): 683, 685.
[54] James G. Wakley, "The Germ Theory of Disease," *The Lancet* (15 May 1875): 694–95.

6. EXPERIMENTAL INVESTIGATION AS A FACTOR IN THE DIFFUSION OF LISTERISM

JAMES WAKLEY COULD NOT have been more wrong about how far those who held the germ theory were willing to go to promote their ideology. This was especially true of Louis Pasteur, who authored *Studies on Fermentation* in 1876; that same year Robert Koch, the German physician who later fired the fatal shot at spontaneous generationism when he isolated the tubercle bacillus, hit the mark in his opening foray against it by tracing the complete life cycle of anthrax bacillus. Pasteur's book included an appendix which cited a paper read by John Tyndall to the Royal Society of London on January 13, 1876. In addition, it reprinted the text of a letter from Tyndall to Pasteur dated the sixteenth of the following month.[1]

Before elaborating on Tyndall's written comments to the noted French chemist, it is necessary to deal with the ramifications of the speech that Tyndall delivered at the Royal Society. He insisted that he had followed exactly the same procedure as H. Charlton Bastian for obtaining "putrefaction of some fluids in hermetically sealed vessels from which the air has been expelled by boiling," but that he had failed one-hundred and thirty-nine times. Predictably, Bastian was the one who replied to Tyndall's latest researches, describing them as founded on "lack of learning and want of attention to prescribed conditions."

Consequently, Tyndall now affirmed that germs were destroyed after five minutes of boiling, to which Bastian responded that "nothing remains but for us to shake hands over the establishment of the occurrence of 'spontaneous generation,' and the overthrow of the Germ Theory of Disease." Tyndall's choice of a five minute waiting period unfortunately played into Bastian's hands, and he "unwittingly . . . became a supporter of Bastian's misplaced confidence in the lethal effect" on microorganisms of continuous boiling. Bastian had specifically advocated a five to ten minute time-frame for the killing of "bacteria and their germs" and sarcastically compared Tyndall to Rip Van Winkle, though he limited Tyndall's sleep to the previous three years. He also chastised Tyndall for not being more attentive to current developments in light of the influence he exerted on the medical profession, which in turn provided health care to the general public.[2]

Obviously chaffing from Bastian's acid pen, Tyndall wrote the editors of *The Times* and *The Lancet,* assuring his readers that he understood the seriousness of propagating his views but pointing out that his adversary had also had great success in publicizing his opinions. He also vented his resentment at Bastian's depiction of Pasteur as "a mere

[1] L. Pasteur, *Studies on Fermentation: The Diseases of Beer, Their Causes, and the Means of Preventing Them* (London: Macmillan & Co., 1879; reprint ed., New York: Kraus Reprint Co., 1969), p. 399; Thomas D. Brock, *Robert Koch: A Life in Medicine and Bacteriology* (Madison, Wisconsin: Science Tech Publishers, 1988), pp. 31–37.
[2] H. Charlton Bastian, "Remarks on a New Attempt to Establish the Truth of the Germ Theory," *The Lancet* (5 February 1876): 206–208; Glenn Vandervliet, *Microbiology and the Spontaneous Generation Debate During the 1870's* (Lawrence, Kansas: Coronado Press, 1971), p. 54.

experimenter" and instead described Pasteur's work as "immortal."[3] Tyndall did not use the same word in his personal correspondence to Pasteur, but he did comment on "the unassailable exactness" of the Frenchman's findings. He mentioned Bastian in his letter too, picturing him as "a young physician" who had "produced an immense impression on the English as well as the American public." Tyndall said that Bastian's books had "made but slight impression on those who know them thoroughly" but that they had "misled" the English people. He felt that his own researches had "refuted many of the errors" contained in them.[4]

Ever combative when it came to defending bacteriology, Pasteur determined to do battle with Bastian himself, especially after the Englishman brashly offered to come to Paris and demonstrate his findings in Pasteur's laboratory at the Ecole Normale Superieure. At approximately the same time he made his proposition, Bastian also submitted an article to the *Contemporary Review* on spontaneous generation, under the pseudonym "Inquirer." He advised Tyndall to forego his earlier experiments and start over, saying that supporters of the germ theory were "not quite agreed as to the answer to be given to the facts advanced by their adversaries."[5] It was during a dialogue with Bastian, which ensued after his proposal, that Pasteur realized for the first time why F. A. Pouchet had achieved results diametrically opposed to his.

Pouchet and Bastian used hay infusions, and Pasteur used yeast water. Cultures made with hay water contained spores of the *bacillus subtilis,* an aerobic bacterium. Its spores remained inactive as long as they were prevented from coming into contact with oxygen, but when oxygen reentered the flask in which the infusions had been heated, they began to develop. After coming to this realization during his tete-a-tete with Bastian, Pasteur customarily increased the temperature for the purpose of sterilization to one-hundred and twenty degrees centigrade. One of the main problems faced by germ theorists was to defend themselves against detractors who argued that their experiments were only "laboratory work" with no clinical application. This was one of the reasons why Pasteur chose to debate Bastian. In July, 1877, he sent Bastian a letter outlining his position and asked him,

> Do you know why I desire so much to fight and conquer you? it [*sic*] is because you are one of the principle adepts of a medical doctrine which I believe to be fatal to progress in the art of healing—the doctrine of the spontaneity of all diseases. . . . That is an error which, I repeat it, is harmful to medical progress. From the prophylactic as well as from the therapeutic point of view, the fate of the physician and surgeon depends upon the adoption of the one or the other of these two doctrines.[6]

Pasteur had already asked the French Academy of Medicine to commission a panel of experts to investigate the question of the germ theory in relation to the disease of

---

[3] John Tyndall, "The Germ Theory," *The Lancet* (12 February 1876): 262.
[4] Pasteur, *Studies on Fermentation,* pp. 400–401.
[5] James G. Wakley, "The Germ Theory and Spontaneous Generation," *The Lancet* (12 May 1877): 691–93.
[6] Rene Vallery-Radot, *The Life of Pasteur* (Garden City, New York: Doubleday, Page & Company, 1926), pp. 253–56.

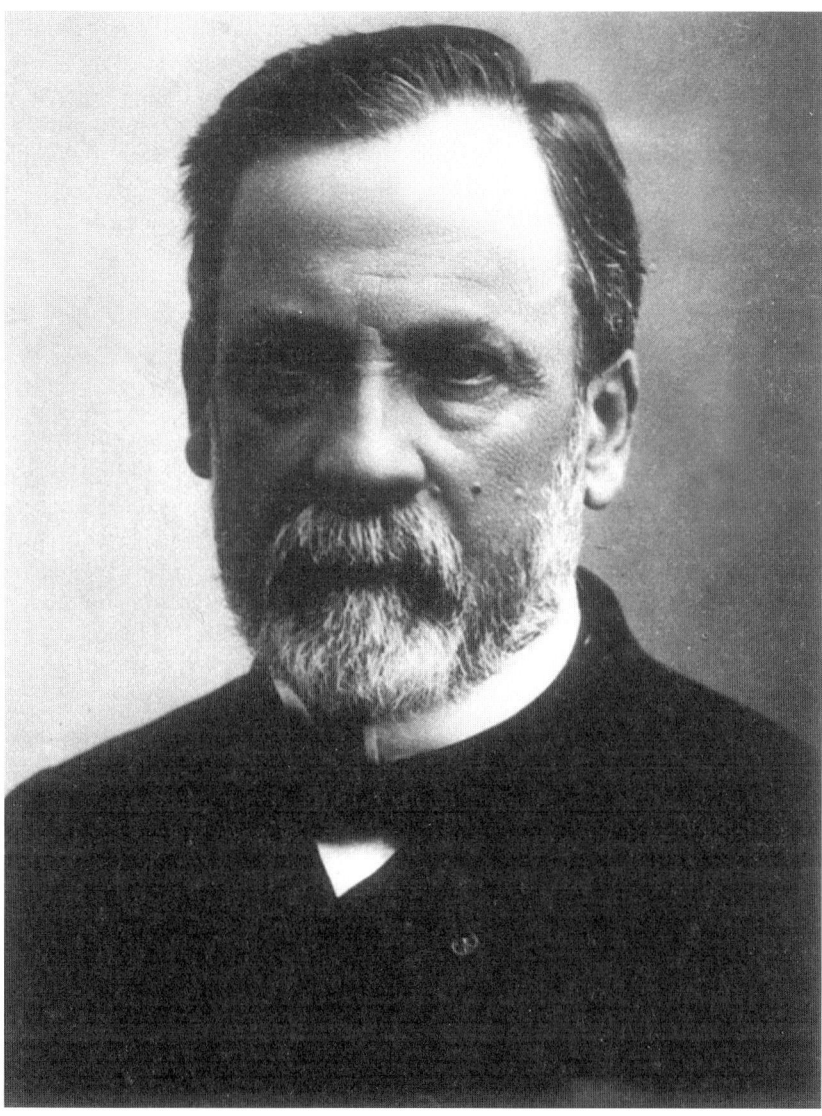

Figure 11. Louis Pasteur

anthrax and make a determination concerning its validity. (See Figure 11.) The committee of five men met on July 20, 1877, and drafted a report that sustained the germ theory. For the first time a direct causal relationship had been established between a specific microorganism and the outbreak of a disease. Just two days before the report of the French Academy of Medicine was drawn up Bastian was at Pasteur's laboratory to demonstrate his procedure in front of a three-man commission appointed by the French Academy of Sciences. Though the arch rivals finally met that day, the commissioners "failed to agree upon the conditions under which the experiments should be conducted," and "the contest between Bastian and Pasteur never did occur."[7]

While Pasteur had been busy preparing for Bastian's visit, Tyndall provided convincing evidence of the germ theory at the Royal Institution. Infusions in both ends of an open rod were heated to the boiling point. One became clear after only five minutes while the other remained clouded with bacteria after fifteen minutes. Tyndall reasoned that it was illogical to explain the phenomenon using the argument of spontaneous generation, since the two culture mediums were in such close proximity, and he submitted that it made no sense for there to be pure air at one end of the rod and infected air at the other. The only explanation that had merit was that the infusions themselves contained germs, some of which were destroyed by boiling and some of which were resistant to that amount of heat.[8]

Tyndall's work on the resistance of germs ultimately clarified why some cultures could not be sterilized with the continuous application of a temperature of one-hundred degrees centigrade; on one occasion microorganisms grew on an infusion after it had been boiled for eight hours. Tyndall advocated the intermittent heating of media to kill resistant germs and maintained that there was a "parallel in the spread of contagious diseases" to the illustration he had provided. The discontinuous boiling of cultures in order to sterilize them became known as Tyndallization, and he considered the process "infallible, however highly infective the surrounding atmosphere may be." It is still utilized to kill "microbial life in egg and serum media and in other heat-sensitive cultivating materials." However, it "is not an effective method of sterilization unless the material under treatment favors spore germination."[9]

Joseph Lister quickly joined Tyndall in his support for Pasteur and his theory. On October 1, 1877, Lister delivered his first lecture as a faculty member at King's College in London, for the opening of its fall medical session. It was entitled "On the Nature of Fermentation," and in it he called putrefaction a "true fermentation" because it was "characterized by the power of self-multiplication of the ferment." Lister defined a ferment as "an active agent" capable of reproducing itself and observed that putrefying blood had the same bacteria as fermenting grape juice. He noted that the microorganisms were labeled bacteria because they were shaped like rods, although they could be of different sizes and were "endowed with a remarkable power of locomotion." The rest of his time was spent proving that they were the cause of the putrefaction and not the result of it. He demonstrated experiments which showed that blood, like infusions of yeast or urine, did not have an "inherent tendency to putrefy" but remained free of contamination in properly sealed containers that were sufficiently heated. Interestingly, he tested this idea further by studying lactic acid and the fermentation of milk, the same experiment Pasteur had used twenty years earlier to initiate his research on the germ theory.[10]

---

[7] Ibid., pp. 276–79; Vandervliet, *Microbiology*, pp. 60–62.

[8] Wakley, "Spontaneous Generation," (16 June 1877): 886; John Tyndall, *Fragments of Science*, 2 vols. (New York: D. Appleton and Company, 1898), 2:290–334.

[9] Ibid; J. K. Crellin, "The Problem of Heat Resistance of Micro-Organisms in the British Spontaneous Generation Controversies of 1860–1880," *Medical History* 10 (January 1966): 56–57; Vandervliet, *Microbiology*, pp. 62–63, 84–85.

[10] Joseph Lister, *The Collected Papers of Joseph, Baron Lister*, 2 vols. (Oxford: The Clarendon Press, 1909), 1:335–41.

Rene Dubos, the best recent biographer of the father of the germ theory, has noted that "the year 1877 constitutes a landmark in the life of Pasteur and in the history of medicine." It was the year that the French chemist finally applied his theory to disease as well as to fermentation, and "the germ theory of disease was accepted in medical circles only after 1877."[11] Indeed, by the end of that year even Wakley wrote that the comparative studies that had been done strongly favored the germ theory. He also cited a new experiment by Tyndall as the most supportive for "evidence of the influence of pure and impure air on the development of bacteria." The eminent physicist had sterilized fifty bottles of assorted infused liquids, after which he had opened twenty-three of them in a hay loft and the others on the ledge of a bluff in the Alps. Twenty-one of the former quickly swarmed with bacteria while none of the latter did. Surely, a scientific revolution was in the making if Wakley sided with the germ theorists and honored Tyndall's research with constructive comments.[12]

Three days after Wakley's remarks appeared, Lister addressed the Pathological Society of London concerning further results of his experiments on the souring of milk. He would no longer be conspicuous by his absence from that illustrious organization, where so much heated debate had occurred, because it elected him to membership that very night. He told his listeners that bacterium lactis was so small that it could only be detected in groups. It was much more minuscule than the granules in yeast that had been the standard for measuring microbes for years. Lister even showed how it diminished with each day that passed until "at last the majority would be so small, and so entangled in the curd, like blood-corpuscles in coagulating fibrin, that they may not be seen." This prompted him to speculate that such diseases as erysipelas were caused by "ultra-microscopical organisms" not visible with the instruments then available, and possibly never to be seen. Most importantly, he had succeeded in procuring the first pure culture of bacteria.[13]

Lister recognized that acceptance of the germ theory was "by no means universal" among physicians and that some physiologists and pathologists still believed bacteria to be "mere accidental concomitants" of fermentation.[14] That is precisely what Bastian said in an article for *The British Medical Journal* published at the beginning of the new year. Although he had admitted that Lister's experiments on the fermentation of milk did not appear to have any flaws in them and that his logic was sound, Bastian acted as if he were unaffected by the irrefutable changes taking place around him. In an incredibly sanguine tone he uttered,

> Thus, all the distinctive positions of those who advocate a belief in the so-called "germ-theory of disease", or rely upon the exclusive doctrine of a "contagium vivum", seem to be absolutely broken down and refuted. We may give that attention to the appearance and development of independent organisms in association with morbid processes which the importance of their presence demands,

[11] Rene Dubos, *Pasteur and Modern Science* (London: Heinemann, 1960), p. 94.
[12] James G. Wakley, "Present State of the Bacteria Question," *The Lancet* (15 December 1877): 893.
[13] James G. Wakley, "Pathological Society of London," *The Lancet* (22 December 1877): 918, 920; Vandervliet, *Microbiology,* p. 17.
[14] Lister, *Collected Papers,* 1:353.

but we must regard them as concomitant products, and not at all, or except to an extremely limited extent, as causes of those local and general diseases with which they are inseparably linked.[15]

John Burdon-Sanderson also composed an article for the same periodical in the first month of 1878, but he showed his sagacity when he ascertained that "bacteria or their germs may exist in the tissues of the animal body without in any way interfering with health."[16] This poignantly illustrates the difference in an intellectually honest seeker of truth and one who has prejudged a matter. Burdon-Sanderson changed his attitude and contributed to the body of knowledge gained in relation to microorganisms. He expressed total agreement with Lister's speech to the London Pathological Society.

By this time Burdon-Sanderson actually had more in common with Lister than he did with Tyndall because Lister taught that bacteria did not come from parent germs already in the body, while Tyndall defined a germ as something that produces a seed. Spores of bacteria had only been discovered in two forms, one of which was *bacillus anthracis,* and this was considered inadequate proof of the presence of seeds for all bacteria by Lister and Burdon-Sanderson. Predictably, Bastian, who did not die until 1915, never renounced the theory of spontaneous generation, "nor did he accept the idea that spores were sufficiently resistant to account for growth in infusions that had been boiled for a short while."[17]

When it became apparent that the germ theorists were winning the day, the distinguished French physiologist, Claude Bernard, struck at the very foundation of Pasteur's research method and postulated that yeast itself could be generated spontaneously. Bernard had discovered that the liver produces glycogen and had elucidated "the function and nature of the vasomotor nerves." He was also one of the first to move medicine from the hospital to the laboratory. Pasteur summarily disposed of Bernard's assumption by returning to one of his most impressive displays of genius. He simply proceeded "to remove with a fine needle the juice from grapes with undamaged skin, and to show that if this was done with all precautions necessary to avoid contact with air or objects, the juice did not ferment until yeast had been added to it."[18] Unlike many other experimenters, Pasteur was always willing to replicate his previous results whenever they were challenged anew.

The evidence in favor of the germ theory of disease was so overwhelming by the end of 1878 that the debate which had raged for a decade in the United Kingdom was reduced to a whisper. Very little can be found on the subject in British medical journals for 1879, and the triumph of germ theorists was made clear when editorial emphasis shifted to a discussion of the nature of disease-causing microorganisms. Robert Koch's studies on pyemia became the topic of much discussion because he had

---

[15] H. Charlton Bastian, "The Bearing of Experimental Evidence upon the Germ-Theory of Disease," *The British Medical Journal* (12 January 1878): 52; Wakley, "Pathological Society," p. 921.

[16] John Burdon-Sanderson, "Lectures on the Infective Processes of Disease," *The British Medical Journal* (26 January 1878): 119.

[17] Wakley, "Pathological Society," pp. 920–21; Crellin, "Heat Resistance," pp. 55, 58.

[18] Dubos, *Pasteur and Modern Science,* p. 56; Erwin H. Ackerknecht, *A Short History of Medicine,* rev. ed. (Baltimore: The Johns Hopkins University Press, 1982), pp. 164, 170.

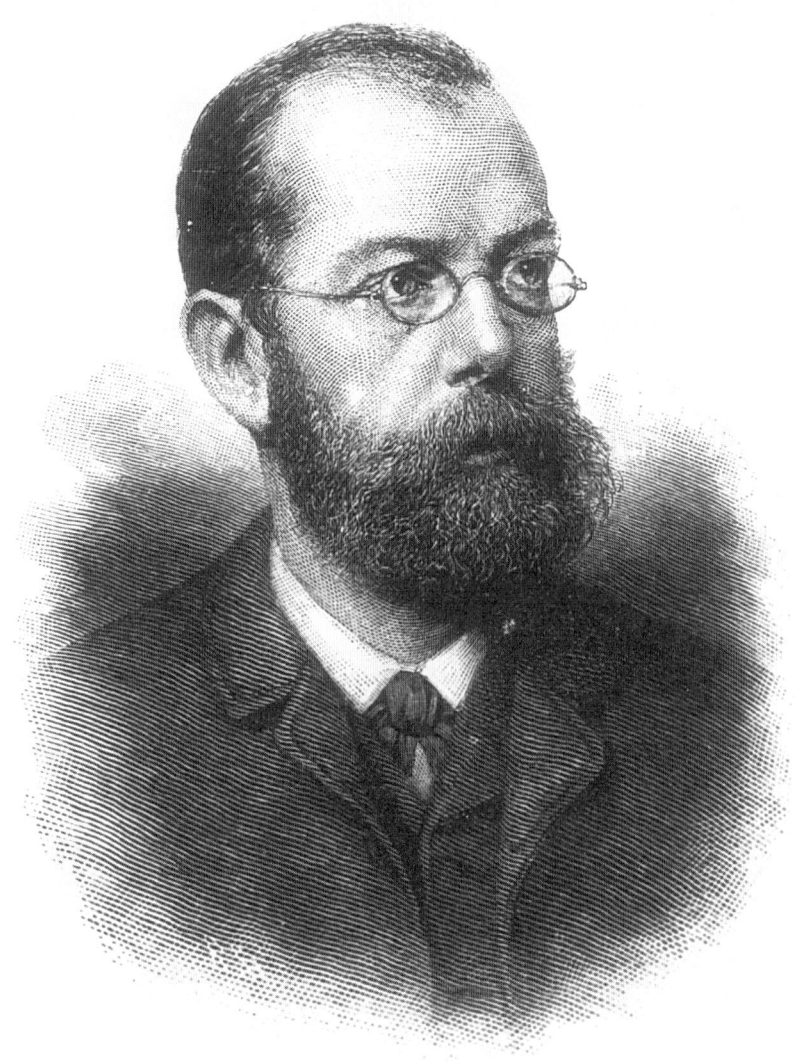

Figure 12. Robert Koch

demonstrated that rabbits got the disease from microorganisms other than those that were rod-shaped. He had found that some micrococci, which were globular or oval bacteria, caused disease, while others produced fermentation.[19] (See Figure 12.)

Koch had also experimented with rabbits to determine the life cycle of anthrax. Obtaining an infected animal hide, he had injected the ear and back of a hare with the diseased matter. That rabbit died in a day, but when a second's corneas were inocu-

---

[19] Wakley, "Pathological Society," (17 May 1879): 703–705.

lated with substance from the first, no sickness occurred. Only when the corneas were cut did it die, giving Koch the "brilliant idea" that anthrax could be artificially cultured in "the aqueous humor" of eyes. The cultures grew the "resting spores" of the disease, but to be sure that it was not transformed as it moved from one host to another, he "passed" a sample of it "through a series of 20 mice." There was no change in the bacteria, which the renowned botanist, Ferdinand Cohn, had already named and classified as a species. Regardless of Koch's fastidiousness, another celebrated researcher, Rudolf Virchow, considered his conclusions "quite improbable." Virchow was Germany's greatest physician and the founder of cellular pathology, but he rejected the part played by microorganisms in disease until Koch isolated the one responsible for tuberculosis in 1882. For a while even after that discovery, Virchow alluded to Koch's find as the "so-called tubercle bacillus." Not all observers were so obstinate, however. Burdon-Sanderson's attitude shift had taken place after a visit to Germany in 1877. Koch had personally showed him active and cultured anthrax.[20]

Koch's work on pyemia was cited by another Englishman, William Watson Cheyne, who argued that the antiseptic technique did not, after all, keep all living organisms from entering a wound; it had precluded the development of rod-shaped bacteria in every case he had witnessed in the previous three years, though. Cheyne had become Lister's house-surgeon in 1876, the year Koch charted the course of anthrax, and had discovered micrococci under carbolic acid dressings. He not only knew that there were many types of microbes but also thought that "it is quite certain that if there are noxious forms of micrococci, they are rare, and that the conditions which allow of the entrance of ordinary forms to wounds treated antiseptically do not admit of the entrance of hurtful kinds." Furthermore, Cheyne went on record against spontaneous generation, saying that it had been so discredited that it was essentially a waste of time to discuss it. Cheyne's comments were made at a meeting of the Pathological Society of London, and Lister was given a chance to respond. He confessed that Cheyne's findings were "unexpected," but plainly stated that in those cases where bacteria had appeared under carbolic-acid dressings it was "from imperfect application of antiseptics." He concluded his remarks by expressing the hope that the day would come when "some more perfect means might be found whereby all organisms could be excluded."[21]

In relating the details of the meeting of the Pathological Society, Wakley editorialized that Lister's method had not been dealt as severe a blow by Cheyne's research as some might think. On the contrary, carbolic acid had been shown to be all the more effective as a bactericide, leading Wakley to conclude that the true "test of thorough antisepticism rests, then, no longer upon the absence of organisms from discharges, but upon that of a special form—the bacterium."[22] Wakley's comments were made in January, 1880, and seven months later Lister spoke to the pathological section of the British Medical Association on the relationship between microorganisms and disease.

The Association met in Cambridge that year, and Lister paid homage to Koch,

---

[20] Brock, *Robert Koch*, pp. 11, 29, 32–33, 38, 71–72, 81–82, 126–27, 132, 136–37; Lois Magner, *A History of Medicine* (New York: Marcel Dekker, Inc., 1992), pp. 316–321.
[21] Wakley, "Pathological Society," (17 May 1879): 703–705.
[22] James G. Wakley, "Organisms Under Antiseptic Dressings," *The Lancet* (17 May 1879): 710–11.

who had formulated ways to stain bacteria, and to Pasteur, who had attenuated the virus responsible for chicken cholera. As one whose father had contributed so much to microscopical science, Lister was especially appreciative of the coloring of germs by the "hard-worked general practitioner" from Germany; Koch had made them "discernible by the human eye." Joseph Jackson Lister had invented an achromatic lens that reduced opalescence and obfuscation so that extremely small objects could be viewed in white light. It transmitted such light without producing the various colors of the spectrum. For his efforts, the elder Lister was admitted to the Royal Society in 1832.[23]

Koch had been able to exhibit the presence of the anthrax bacillus in the blood of the smallest vessels of the body, not just the spleen and other major organs. He also hypothesized that septicemia was a blood disease due to microorganisms and that it was "equally distinct from pyaemia and from the chemically toxic effects of septic products." Two other diseases considered particularly grievous by physicians, gangrene and erysipelas, were associated with specific germs by Koch, though it was Friedrich Fehleisen who finally isolated the latter in 1883. Truly, an explosion of knowledge was accompanying the reception of Pasteur's germ theory of disease by the medical profession. Practitioners embraced it as suddenly as they had renounced it, once the evidence for it came rushing in with the assistance of men like Koch.[24]

Changing his subject to Pasteur, Lister pointed out that the legendary French chemist had isolated the microbe responsible for cholera in chickens and had cultivated it "outside the body of the fowl." Pasteur was then able to weaken its potency and make a vaccine from it. When chickens were vaccinated with the attenuated virus, they became immune to the disease. The same procedure was also shown to be effective in providing cattle with immunity to anthrax. Lister was so optimistic about the future that he dared to envision the possible consequences of a renewed interest in vaccinations. Limiting his scope to the next decade, he ventured,

> I need hardly remark on the surpassing importance of researches such as these. No one can say but that, if the British Medical Association should meet at Cambridge again ten years hence, some one may be able to record the discovery of the appropriate vaccine for measles, scarlet fever, and other acute specific diseases of the human subject. But even should nothing more be effected than what seems to be already on the point of attainment . . . it must be admitted that we have here an instance of a most valuable result from the much-reviled vivisection.[25]

Unfortunately, a vaccine for measles had to wait longer than a decade, and scarlet fever was not treated effectively until the discovery of penicillin. The latter reached epidemic proportions in Britain during Lister's career, and was the leading cause of death in children; ninety-five percent of those who contracted the disease were

---

[23] Lister, *Collected Papers*, 1:387, 390; 2:543–52; Richard B. Fisher, *Joseph Lister, 1827–1912* (New York: Stein and Day, 1977), p. 21.
[24] Lister, *Collected Papers*, 1:387–90; Ackerknecht, *Short History*, p. 180.
[25] Lister, *Collected Papers*, 1:390–92, 394.

younger than ten. Thirty-four thousand had perished with it in 1863, and more than twenty-six thousand more expired in 1874. "As late as the 1880s in Edinburgh about one child died for every fourteen catching the disease, while in the great epidemic of 1880 it carried off almost one child in five who contracted it." In spite of these incidences of extremely high death tolls, though, the overall percentage of mortality from the disease dropped eighty-one points from 1861 to 1891.[26]

Still, by comparison scarlet fever continued to be a much feared ailment. For instance, from 1865 to 1894 the Glasgow Fever Hospital had twice as many cases of it as other diseases, with a mortality rate of approximately ten percent. A higher percentage died from typhus and typhoid fever, which were second and third on the list, respectively. Measles was fourth and resulted in slightly less than nine percent fatalities. Many of the "acute specific diseases of the human subject" mentioned by Lister were traced to microorganisms during the period foreseen. They included typhoid fever, leprosy, malaria, tuberculosis, glanders, erysipelas, cholera, diphtheria, tetanus, pneumonia, epidemic meningitis, undulant fever, and soft chancre.[27]

Also, a short eight months after Lister's speech Wakley recorded that doubts about the germ theory no longer captured the imagination of the medical community because it had been repeatedly shown to be true. In other words, hardly anyone questioned what had been the most controversial topic of the dozen previous years in Great Britain. Wakley also gave Lister what the latter must have considered to be the ultimate compliment when he said that "no longer the recognised novelty, 'Listerism' has become the recognised necessity of civilised surgery, for the voice of the surgical world proclaims its truth." In a manner that surely seemed to Lister to have erased years of doubt about his technique, Wakley then asked his readers, "And what is antiseptic surgery but the rational application of the germ theory?"[28] Suddenly, as if blinders had been lifted from his eyes, Wakley could see a logical connection between the germ theory and disease, and in the next decade he and other die-hards witnessed an explosion in associating specific diseases with particular germs.

Of all the illnesses so linked between 1880 and 1890, the most devastating was tuberculosis, and developing a way to diagnose it made Koch famous. In England, Koch was kept before the medical profession by George Harley who authored a three-part article for *The Lancet* in June, 1881, entitled "Etiology and Clinical Bearings of the Germ Theory of Disease." Harley, a fellow of the Royal Society, alluded to the aniline dye used by Koch to color bacteria and gave insight into the early stages of experimentation on tuberculosis. He related that animals on the Continent had been inoculated with the tubercle bacillus, which "produced tuberculous deposits."[29] He also divulged that Koch had demonstrated a connection between abscesses and streptococci as well as the role of microorganisms in the formation of embolus. These suc-

[26] Anthony S. Wohl, *Endangered Lives: Public Health in Victorian Britain* (Cambridge, Massachusetts: Harvard University Press, 1983), pp. 128–29.
[27] Olive Checkland, "Local government and the health environment," in *Health Care as Social History: The Glasgow Case*, ed. Olive Checkland and Margaret Lamb (Aberdeen, Scotland: Aberdeen University Press, 1982), p. 12; Ackerknecht, *Short History*, p. 180.
[28] James G. Wakley, "'Blood Diseases' and the 'Germ Theory'," *The Lancet* (2 April 1881): 546–47.
[29] George Harley, "Etiology and Clinical Bearings of the Germ Theory of Disease," *The Lancet* (4 June 1881): 903, 907; Koch used methyl violet more than the other aniline dyes, but they all "permitted distinction of bacteria from nonliving precipitates, fat droplets, or other tiny bodies." Brock, *Robert Koch*, p. 63.

cesses led Harley to hope that every infectious and contagious disease might be tied to specific germs.[30]

Utilizing a set of postulates recommended by Koch, researchers were able to link many bacteria with the particular illnesses they caused. His guidelines involved finding the germ in each occurrence of a certain disease, making sure it was not found in any other ailment, isolating it, culturing it, inoculating it to see if it produced the same sickness, and recovering it from the animal that had been inoculated. Koch had suggested these rules in his book, *Aetiology of Traumatic Infective Diseases,* which was published in 1878; today, they are collectively stated as three postulates.[31] Cheyne considered this book so important that he translated it for publication by the New Sydenham Society two years later. Koch also demolished the theory of polymorphism, which said that germs were able to modify themselves into new forms. Those who tried to justify their inability to secure pure bacterial cultures held this view.[32]

The triumph of bacteriology was completed at the 1881 International Medical Congress, which was held in London. Both Lister and Pasteur delivered major speeches. When Bastian created a controversy during the discussion of Lister's paper by bringing up the idea of heterogenesis, Pasteur was unable to remain silent. "Mais, mon Dieu," he shouted, while using his fist to strike the table, "ce n'est pas possible— jamais, jamais." Lister had noted that Koch was present at the meeting, praised his work, and told the assembled physicians that the German surgeon had agreed to demonstrate his technique at King's College. Lister had also affirmed that he considered the evidence presented by Koch to be confirmation of his observations on microorganisms and their relationship to disease.[33]

If Lister's speech dealt with Koch and his findings, Pasteur's did not. He ignored the German physician but paid tribute to Lister, calling him a "great surgeon." He also talked about "the lively feeling of satisfaction" he enjoyed when Lister announced that his 1857 publication on the fermentation of milk was the inspiration for antisepsis. More pertinently, Pasteur disclosed his opinion that oxygen acts as a modifier of bacteria by making them less virulent. Before concluding his brief remarks, he even explained how earthworms transport the anthrax bacillus from animal graveyards to the top of the ground where other beasts consume them.[34] In his commentary on the International Medical Congress, Wakley shared some of what Koch displayed for the leading medical men in London. He reviewed Koch's experiments on polymorphism, which plainly exhibited that when bacteria are grown on something firm, "such as gelatine, where they could not mix with each other, the numerous varieties could be separated, and kept separate from each other, and that they never underwent any change in form or transformation into each other."[35]

Less than a year after he visited London, Koch became a household name in the

---

[30] Harley, "Etiology," (11 June 1881): 948.
[31] K. Codell Carter, trans., *Essays of Robert Koch* (New York: Greenwood Press, 1987), pp. xiv, xviii, 19–56; Ackerknecht, *Short History,* p. 179.
[32] W. Watson Cheyne, *Lister and His Achievement* (London: Longmans, Green and Co., 1925), pp. 85–87; A. J. Youngson, *The Scientific Revolution in Victorian Medicine* (New York: Holmes & Meier Publishers, Inc., 1979), p. 207.
[33] Lister, *Collected Papers,* 1:399; Stephen Paget, ed., *Memoirs and Letters of Sir James Paget* (London: Longmans, Green and Co., 1901) pp. 410–11.
[34] "Translation of an Address on the Germ Theory [by Louis Pasteur]," *The Lancet* (13 August 1881): 271–72.
[35] James G. Wakley, "The International Medical Congress," *The Lancet* (13 August 1881): 290–91.

British Isles and the rest of the world. He isolated the microbe that causes tuberculosis, a fact that he revealed for the first time at the Berlin Physiological Society on March 24, 1882; it was not unveiled to physicians because Virchow still "dominated" German medicine and "shunned" Koch. The cultured bacteria did not "form visible colonies" for fourteen days, although most render results in forty-eight hours. Koch's patience was rewarded with proof that one of history's deadliest diseases had a specific origin which could be identified; tuberculosis killed every seventh person in the 1800s, more than cholera or smallpox. When Koch ended his revelation, "there was silence. No applause, no questions, no debate. Those who attended the lecture remembered later the silence, not of boredom or doubt, but of stunned admiration at the brilliant work they had just heard." One physician has pithily described Koch's disclosure as having "an electrifying effect." Two by-products of it were that theorizing and "laboratory experimentation acquired greater esteem."[36]

An article in *The Times* on September 5, 1882, discussed the diffusion of bacteria and included a sentence based on Koch's experiments. It warned that tuberculosis "may be transmitted from one person to another by the air passages" and advised caution in regard to contact with the young because millions of bacteria "are found in the dejections of healthy children." It also apprised people of the dangers associated with infectious germs, noting that they multiply on mucous membranes "to a formidable extent" but conceding that their development "on normal mucous surfaces is usually limited."[37] By the end of 1882 Wakley evaluated the tangible benefits of the medical advances experienced since the advent of bacteriology and immunology. He vented the frustration that many physicians felt when they encountered difficulty translating the experimental results into improved health care. He began by placing the research of men like Pasteur and Koch in historical perspective:

> Far be it from us to undervalue the remarkable facts of the relation of living organisms to disease, which have been ascertained by the not less remarkable investigations of the recent years. Their profound importance is beyond all question, and they will certainly constitute a chief landmark of the progress of medical science in the present century. But in the profession, and even more outside it, there has been, and still is, a widespread expectation of practical results of the highest importance from these discoveries—an expectation of an immediate and vast increase in our power of dealing with disease, of preventing its occurrence, and of curing it when it has developed. A caution is needed against such exaggerated expectation.[38]

Even when Koch developed tuberculin from a glycerin extract of cultured tubercle bacillus in 1890, it did not turn out to be the panacea hoped for by the medical profession; it did make it possible to diagnose the disease, however. Lister took his niece to Germany that year but "had to wait a week" for her to be treated because of

---

[36] Magner, *History of Medicine,* pp. 318–21; Brock, *Robert Koch,* pp. 126–32; Lester S. King, "Germ Theory and Its Influence," *The Journal of the American Medical Association* 249 (11 February 1983): 796.

[37] *The Times* (London), 5 September 1882.

[38] James G. Wakley, "Bacterial Pathology," *The Lancet* (2 December 1882): 947.

the attention Koch was receiving.[39] The answers practitioners wanted were still primarily to be found in antisepsis and its evolutionary descendant, asepsis. Only by combining the work of Lister, Pasteur, and Koch would physicians be able to provide maximal protection against the maladies of the day. However, the need for additional in-depth study of diseases would always remain, and the psyche of Victorian perfectionism would have to adjust to that fact.

---

[39] Magner, *History of Medicine*, pp. 321–24; Brock, *Robert Koch*, pp. 209–212.

7. TECHNICAL EVOLUTION AS A FACTOR IN THE DIFFUSION OF LISTERISM

IT MAY HAVE BEEN A QUEST for perfection that drove Joseph Lister to constantly improve his system, but it was definitely a determination to accept nothing less from him that spurred on his opponents. In that vein, yet another article pertaining to the antiseptic treatment of wounds was published in *The Lancet* on January 3, 1874. Its author was Sampson Gamgee, the same special correspondent for the weekly who had reported the difference in how Parisian surgeons and Lister administered carbolic acid seven years earlier. A surgeon at The Queen's Hospital in Birmingham, he was now employed to investigate the day-to-day routine associated with Lister's technique. Gamgee had attended medical school with Lister and considered him a friend. In a two-part commentary, based on an examination of Lister's wards at Edinburgh in December, 1873, he described the theory behind Lister's practice and the intricacies of the practice itself.

Lister trusted Gamgee and had urged him to take notes so that he could offer constructive criticism rather than simply playing the role of a silent visitor. Lister was certain of his ability to persuade Gamgee of the efficacy of his system, and assumed that Gamgee would wholeheartedly endorse it. However, Gamgee took a much more critical view of the antiseptic procedure than Lister had expected. He began by observing that as of 1873 Lister's "counsel" had not as yet won "very general assent," but "that the complacent calmness of supposed orthodoxy" had been "finally disturbed by the heretic blast sounded in Professor Lister's clinique."[1] Pointing out that Lister had repeatedly changed his mind about the form of carbolic acid that should be used in wound management, Gamgee seemed to be perplexed at his tenacity in holding on to Pasteur's doctrine. Specifically, he noted that Lister had foregone the use of full-strength carbolic acid, carbolized oil, and the putty made with the substance. He found Lister's desire to experiment with different agents refreshing but could not understand his obsession with the germ theory. To Gamgee, such a fixation showed that his subject was guilty of "the fatal bias of a fixed theoretical preoccupation."[2]

Gamgee did applaud Lister's procedure for draining wounds but expressed his concern that other "remedial principles" such as suspension and compression were being overlooked. He was also disturbed that Lister did not "weigh the relative advantages of moist and dry, of frequent and rare dressings, with and without drainage." Lister responded to Gamgee's article more defensively than he probably should have if he wanted to influence others through the medical press. Calling Gamgee's assertion that he was preoccupied with theory instead of practice a "grave charge," he implored readers of *The Lancet* to delineate "between the facts which Mr. Gamgee has recorded, and his comments upon them."[3]

---

[1] Sampson Gamgee, "The Treatment of Wounds on the Antiseptic Method," *The Lancet* (3 January 1874): 9.
[2] Ibid., (10 January 1874): 51.
[3] Ibid; Joseph Lister, "Mr. Gamgee's Report on Antiseptic Surgery," *The Lancet* (17 January 1874): 109.

Gamgee retorted that Lister had proofread both sections of his rough draft, correcting the first one but leaving the second one untouched. All of the changes were implemented, but Gamgee's critical statement concerning Lister's "fatal bias" had been added to the second half of the final draft after Lister had seen it. Still, Gamgee did not feel that he had leveled a personal attack on Lister. He insisted, instead, that what he had done was affirm "in the broadest terms, a real want of cotemporary [sic] scientific surgery." Lister obviously felt that his surgery was based on the latest scientific principles.[4] Never one to miss an opportunity to have the last word, Lister replied by saying that he had been given strict instructions not to alter anything other than factual errors, and that it would have been inappropriate for him to have suggested revisions in Gamgee's summation.[5]

Gamgee's conclusion that Lister was solely faithful to the germ theory as the premise for his method was substantiated in a message Lister sent to Pasteur in February. It contained one especially telling sentence in which Lister expressed his gratitude to Pasteur "for having, by your brilliant researches, demonstrated to me the truth of the germ theory of putrefaction, and thus furnished me with the principle upon which alone the antiseptic system can be carried out."[6] Pasteur had a mutual admiration for Lister, expressing his "highest esteem and devotion" for him and his amazement at Lister's "complete understanding of the experimental method." He urged him to send the Academy of Sciences "a rather detailed notice" explaining his technique because French surgeons, in Pasteur's opinion, had "only an incomplete knowledge on this subject."[7]

Since most members of the medical profession in Great Britain did not understand the germ theory and its place in Lister's thought and practice, the main debate among surgeons there focused on Lister's method alone and the ways in which he implemented the antiseptic principle. The overriding issue after 1873 was Lister's use of a carbolic-acid spray and the extent to which it worked. As has been mentioned, Lister tried agents other than carbolic acid as antiseptics, but he did not find them to be nearly as effective. The discussion of Lister's system, therefore, kept coming back to the value of the carbolic-acid spray and his insistence that it killed airborne microorganisms. The controversy surrounding the carbolic-acid spray was directly related to the conflict caused by Pasteur's theory, even though it was often obscured.

Lister had initially revealed his use of a spray on New Year's Eve, 1870, but it gained widespread attention in 1874 due to Gamgee's report and Lister's announcement that he was having a new apparatus built to produce a totally antiseptic atmosphere. Since Lister based his system on saturating the air surrounding a surgical incision with a fine mist of carbolic acid, the announcement of a steam-powered sprayer that "was self-acting and self-directing" was hailed by his supporters. Prior to its introduction, Lister had used manual sprayers, at first worked by hand and then by foot, that necessitated the hiring of "a special skilled assistant, both during the performance of the operation and in changing the dressings." Lister's opponents agreed with the

---

[4] Sampson Gamgee, "Mr. Gamgee's Report on Antiseptic Surgery," *The Lancet* (24 January 1874): 143.
[5] Lister, "Mr. Gamgee's Report," (31 January 1874): 182.
[6] Rene Dubos, *Pasteur and Modern Science* (London: Heinemann, 1960), pp. 99–100.
[7] Louis Pasteur to Joseph Lister, 27 February 1874, (photocopy), Western Manuscripts, Wellcome Institute for the History of Medicine, London, MS 69/0, 11.

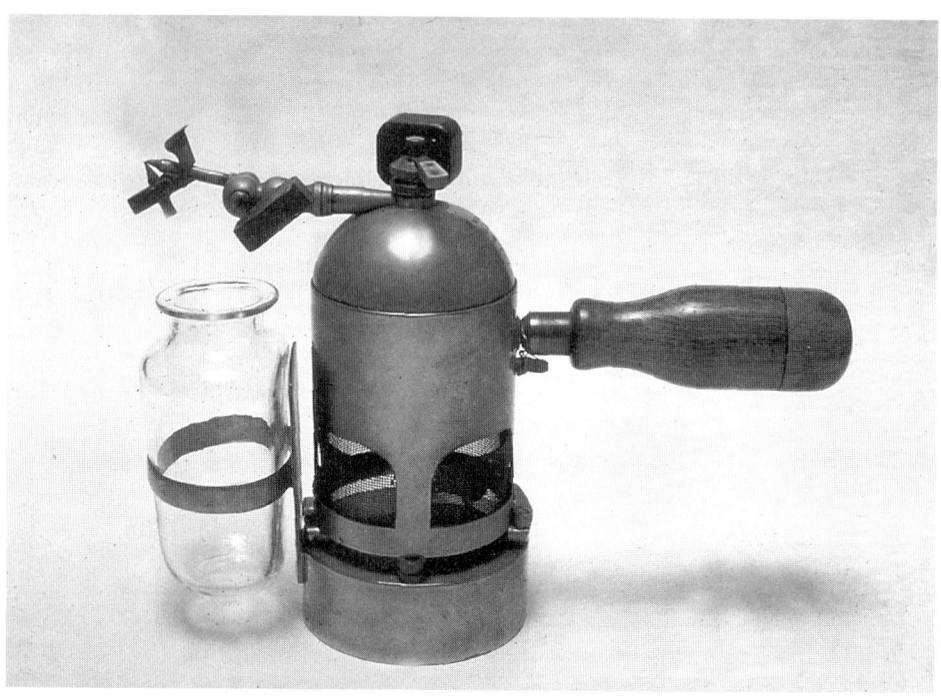

Figure 13. Steam Sprayer

general perception that the spray was the "weak point" of the antiseptic system, and even those who adhered to Lister's principle doubted the necessity of permeating operating rooms with it.[8] (See Figure 13.)

In addition to spraying carbolic acid throughout the surgical environment, Lister introduced the British medical profession to other innovations for combating sepsis. The September, 1874, edition of the *Edinburgh Medical Journal* contained a communication by Lister to the Scottish capital's Medico-Chirurgical Society on a new antiseptic that he considered suitable for use in treating epithelial ulcers. The substance was boric acid, which was less irritating than carbolic acid and, consequently, did not have to have a protective layer of cloth separating it from such surfaces as facial tissues. This was of the utmost importance because putrefaction occurred extremely easily in places like the mouth and nostrils. One member of the society was particularly impressed by this new agent because it promised to be advantageous not only for surgeons but also for physicians, who dealt more with general medicine.[9]

---

[8] Carbolic-acid sprayers consisted of two connected tubes, one through which air was forced to draw the liquid through the other one; the concentration of the liquid had to be greater for a steam machine because of the additional dilution that occurred; more than one sprayer was often required to create an antiseptic cloud in the operating room, unless several connected tubes were used in a single machine for convenience; Lister's steam-powered sprayer had a capacity that could last roughly two hours, but other problems arose such as clogged orifices, especially since they were made extremely small to produce the finest mist possible. Just Lucas-Championniere, *Antiseptic Surgery: The Principles, Modes of Application, and Results of the Lister Dressing* (Portland, Maine: Loring, Short, and Harmon, 1881), pp. 75–77; William Craig, "Medico-Chirurgical Society of Edinburgh," *Edinburgh Medical Journal* 20 (July 1874): 72–73.
[9] Craig, "Medico-Chirurgical," (September 1874): 268–70.

Thus, even when Lister's other innovations were well received, critics would still attack him because of his reliance on the spray. This was not only true of his fellow countrymen but also of some French practitioners. The latter occasionally attempted to refute Lister in an effort to attack Pasteur indirectly, who was gaining too much popularity to suit them. One such opponent of Lister in France was M. Demarquay whose "Note on the Carbolic Acid Mode of Dressing Wounds (Lister's Process), and on the Development of Vibrios in the Wounds" was published by the *Gazette Medicale de Paris* in 1874. Demarquay was against the use of carbolic acid in any form, but especially as a spray for disinfecting the air. He actually stated that when the mist hit the wound it promoted bleeding, caused difficulty in determining the amount of blood lost, and made bleeding harder to stop. More specifically, he accused it of thinning the blood so that it took longer to coagulate, and he categorically asserted that it "encouraged haemorrhage." Finally, Demarquay dogmatically declared "that operative procedures or dressings in a hospital are powerless to prevent or arrest the development of vibrios."[10] His comments were obviously directed as much to Pasteur as to Lister, but he was clearly reckless in his charge that carbolic acid retarded coagulation because experiments dealing with its action on albumin had shown just the opposite to be true. Indeed, "its coagulating power has been, perhaps, over estimated."[11]

Lister needed support for the spray, and it came from an unlikely place. A surgeon at Guy's Hospital in London, the city where Lister's innovations were resisted the most, defended the use of carbolic-acid spray. His testimony was all the more crucial because he operated on the abdomen. Abdominal surgery was particularly life-threatening, and not coincidentally, many of Lister's antagonists were those who opened the peritoneal cavity. However, this practitioner was of the opinion that the spray facilitated surgical procedures on the viscera, as long as certain safeguards were followed. He cautioned that the vapor should not come into contact with exposed intestines and that an attendant should be ready at all times to drape a cloth over any that were. He did acknowledge that the acid caused irritation, and in cases where a patient was debilitated could prove to be dangerous, but he candidly admitted that "this risk is not in the slightest degree comparable to that which is caused by the introduction of septic materials from without."[12]

The same sentiment was stated by William Macewen, who served as casualty surgeon at the dispensary of the Glasgow Royal Infirmary. His specialty was thoracic surgery, and he applauded antisepticism because it allowed him to examine penetrating wounds of the chest cavity with either a probe or his finger. Noting the fact that one-hundred and twenty out of one-hundred and forty-seven British soldiers who received such injuries during the Crimean War died, he chronicled what he considered to be an "advance in surgery." He wrote that it was made possible by the use of antiseptics and expressed his preference for Lister's "intelligent treatment" to "groping in the dark."[13]

---

[10] William Craig, "Periscope," *Edinburgh Medical Journal* 20 (November 1874): 463–64.
[11] Arthur Ernest Sansom, *The Antiseptic System: A Treatise on Carbolic Acid and Its Compounds* (Philadelphia: J. B. Lippincott and Co., 1871), p. 11.
[12] H. G. Howse, "Two Cases of Internal Intestinal Obstruction Treated by Operation," *Guy's Hospital Reports,* Third Series, 19 (1874): 504–505.
[13] William Macewen, "Penetrating Wounds of Thorax and Abdomen Treated Antiseptically," *The Glasgow Medical Journal,* n.s., 7 (January 1875): 6.

Not all Glaswegian surgeons agreed with Macewen, in part because they had not seen tangible proof of the advantages of the antiseptic system. One surgeon who performed operations on the intestinal tract clearly had been led to expect too much. He had understood that there would be no drainage in wounds treated antiseptically, including sanguineous as well as purulent discharge. In addition, he chose to replace the intestines and simply suture the wound instead of applying an antiseptic that would irritate the site; he did include ligatures made from catgut among those he elected to use. He was criticized by Hector C. Cameron, though, for being "so enthusiastic as to believe that in any treatment where there were divided vessels, there would be no bleeding." Cameron, who had been Lister's house-surgeon in Glasgow, was shocked that anyone would think such a thing when Lister had advised that serous fluids should be allowed to pass from wounds. Cameron also lectured the "enthusiastic" surgeon on the profound difference in regular catgut ligatures and those that were antiseptically prepared.[14]

If some remained wary of Lister's system, others proposed expanding its application. Thomas Annandale, who taught in the same department as Lister at the University of Edinburgh and practiced medicine at the Edinburgh Royal Infirmary, proposed increasing the number of exploratory surgeries in light of the security provided by the antiseptic principle. Such surgeries were very helpful in determining whether or not wounds inflicted to the pelvic cavity were beginning to suppurate, something needles could not always tell the practitioner. They had also aided in assessing the chances for success in the removal of certain growths. Annandale had even used incision to remove pus from diseased joints and to diagnose bone injuries as either dislocations or fractures. Finally, he added intestinal obstructions and kidney stones to his list of ailments that could be relieved by exploratory measures.[15]

Undoubtedly aware of the heightened interest in the progress of his technique, Lister decided to write a detailed article on the most recent improvements that he and others had made. This seven-part series appeared in *The Lancet* between March and June, 1875, and described the course of the antiseptic system since Lister's address in surgery at the Plymouth conference of the British Medical Association four years earlier. Lister had settled on a solution of one part carbolic acid to twenty parts water before surgery to prepare the skin of the patient, to cleanse instruments and sponges, and "for washing accidental wounds so as to destroy once for all any septic organisms that may have been introduced into them." Furthermore, he maintained that antiseptic gauzes were still "trustworthy if properly used," which meant applying them in eight layers with an additional sheet of an impermeable material like mackintosh that was

> placed beneath the outermost layer to prevent the discharge from soaking directly through the dressing, for if it did so a copious effusion might wash out the antiseptic from the part immediately over the wound and putrefy within twenty-four hours.[16]

[14] Joseph Coats, "Transactions of the Medico-Chirurgical Society," *The Glasgow Medical Journal,* n.s., 7 (January 1875): 116.
[15] Thomas Annandale, "Antiseptic Incisions an aid to Surgical Diagnosis," *Edinburgh Medical Journal* 20 (January 1875): 612–15, 617.
[16] Joseph Lister, "On Recent Improvements in the Details of Antiseptic Surgery," *The Lancet* (13 March 1875): 365–66.

In regard to the spray, Lister observed that the use of gauzes would often have proved unsuccessful without it because it "plays on the under surface of the gauze when applied." Otherwise, germs from the air, which attached to the gauzes before they could be positioned in place, remained septic because the carbolic acid contained in the resin of the gauzes was released too slowly to kill them. Lister did not say, however, that the mist from the spray was adequate for the prevention of infection. Either the layer of gauze touching the wound had to be resoaked in a one-to-forty dilution of the acid or an additional piece of cloth, similarly prepared, had to be put between the wound and the eight-layered bandage. Lister recognized that his process was not promoted in many hospitals because it was extremely expensive. Consequently, he reminded surgeons that the gauzes could be boiled and reused in order to save money.[17]

Increasingly conscious of the fact that carbolic acid was not universally effective in all surgical procedures, Lister showed his flexibility by advocating the employment of zinc chloride for treating damaged sinuses in the various parts of the body. His experience had been that one application of it worked for days instead of hours, did not cause tissues to die, and produced "no odour from first to last."[18] An eight and a half percent watery solution of it was used on cut surfaces and could often be left until granulation neared completion. It also stopped substances in the wound from being absorbed by the body.[19] Lister continued to work carbolic acid into as many of his daily procedures as possible, though. He mixed it with oil to lubricate catheters, for example, but finally stated that in cases where suppuration already existed his system was "calculated to prevent, not to correct, putrefaction." This helped put his principle in perspective because those who employed his method could easily lead themselves to believe that performing the intricacies of his technique would reverse infection instead of merely controlling its spread.[20]

Of the many complex aspects of Lister's system, the one that had remained the most painstaking was the insertion of drainage tubes in wounds. Made from India rubber, they varied in thickness from that "of a crow-quill to that of the little finger," and their openings were half the width of the tubes themselves. Lister left them in wounds for three or four days and determined that overstating their significance was not possible. Nevertheless, while he was discussing their use, he was unable to resist the opportunity to try to impose the spray on a skeptical medical profession. He cunningly warned that it ought to "be fairly directed on the wound during the withdrawal of a drainage-tube, the place of which must necessarily be taken by air, which, if not purified by the spray, will be likely to be septic."[21]

Another of Lister's innovations, revealed for the first time in his article and developed to accommodate his practice of using drainage tubes, was the "sinus-forceps." They had been given that name by those in Edinburgh who made instruments. In

---

[17] Ibid., pp. 366–67.
[18] Ibid., (20 March 1875): 401–402.
[19] W. Watson Cheyne, *Manual of the Antiseptic Treatment of Wounds for Students and Practitioners* (New York: J. H. Vail & Co., 1885), p. 126.
[20] Lister, "Recent Improvements," (20 March 1875): 401–402.
[21] Ibid., (27 March 1875): 434–35; J. G. Bonnin and W. R. LeFanu, "Joseph Lister, 1827–1912: A Bibliographical Biography," *The Journal of Bone and Joint Surgery* 49B (February 1967): 12.

actuality, they were ordinary dressing scissors, the blades of which had been "ground down to the size of a probe at their extremities . . . so that they can be passed into a very small orifice." Their practicality in placing drainage tubes in abscesses and other injuries was highly regarded by Lister, and in the midst of his remarks, he took the opportunity to proclaim that if the antiseptic method "had done nothing more than create such a revolution in the treatment of abscess and throw such light upon its pathology, it would have well deserved the gratitude of the surgeon."

By 1875 the extent to which he had shaken the foundations of British medicine had finally dawned on Lister, and his confidence bordered on recklessness. In April, he told his fellow surgeons not to worry if used sponges that had been washed and treated with carbolic acid still had the smell of pus on them from a previous operation. He explained that the "presence of a little of the *products* of putrefaction will do no harm if the *causes* of the fermentation have been destroyed." He also contended that what remained in sponges that had been repeatedly rinsed were solid particles of living organisms that had been divested of their potency, not chemical ferments in solution. The latter would have caused mischief in wounds, in spite of being treated with carbolic acid, whereas the former did not. Lister considered this "to be a sure and important step in proof of the theory upon which the antiseptic treatment is based."[22]

The last three sections of Lister's article focused on the capabilities of boric acid, which he had commented on at the Edinburgh Medico-Chirurgical Society. He had learned about the new antiseptic from a Norwegian friend three years earlier. He told Lister that it was being tested in Sweden, where it had been discovered, to preserve food as well as treat wounds. Lister knew, shortly after applying it to his own ingrown fingernail, that it worked well when utilized as a watery solution on superficial injuries. It would not be sufficient in that form, however, "for a permanent antiseptic dressing under circumstances where there is at all a free discharge."[23]

To make boric acid suitable for more extensive surgical procedures Lister boiled it and put lint in it to absorb as much of the concentrated antiseptic as possible. The lint was then dried, after which it was twice as heavy as normal because of the boric acid crystals that had formed in it. The end product was even better than he anticipated because the crystals, which were "soft and unctuous," were not abrasive to the skin like most other crystallized substances. This made the "boracic lint" especially effective in covering wounds that were due to the complications of simple fractures, in dressing deep burns, and in grafting skin.[24]

Although Lister's stature was growing in Great Britain in the mid-1870s, German surgeons provided the greatest accolades he had yet received. Even Wakley was impressed and described German adoption of Lister's method to his readers. Richard von Volkmann, a surgeon and a teacher at the University of Halle who specialized in osteotomy, said that successful results in such operations could be guaranteed with Lister's technique. Ten of the thirteen patients on whom he had performed bone surgery in 1874 experienced no suppuration, and the other three manifested "only the

---

[22] Lister, "Recent Improvements," (3 April 1875): 468–70.
[23] Ibid., (1 May 1875): 603–604.
[24] Ibid., pp. 604–605; Bonnin and LeFanu, "Joseph Lister," p. 12.

most trifling amount." Also, there had been no fatalities in thirty-one cases of compound fractures and no cases of pyemia in the previous eighteen months, even though sixty major amputations had been carried out during that same period. Wakley concluded that the German professor's findings "deserve the widest publicity—for criticism, if they can be challenged in any way, for imitation if they cannot."[25]

Volkmann was by no means the only German to endorse Lister's principle. On the contrary, at the Congress of German Surgery, which met in Berlin in April of 1875, the "stream of praise became a torrent." Lister was even invited by its members to visit Germany and to see firsthand the kind of results achieved with his method there. He accepted the invitation and toured the cities of Munich, Leipzig, and Berlin, each of which welcomed him like a conquering hero. The Germans remembered Lister's advice concerning the care of wounded soldiers during the Franco-Prussian War and gladly showed their appreciation for his contribution to their military heritage.[26]

A dinner was held in Lister's honor at Munich, and some seventy guests attended. He was introduced by Johann von Nussbaum, a surgeon who had sent his assistant to Edinburgh the year before to learn the antiseptic technique. Nussbaum had nothing but respect and gratitude for Lister. He heartily sanctioned Lister's approach. "Look now at my sick wards recently ravaged by death," he said. "I can only say that I and my assistants and my nurses are over-whelmed with joy and undertake all the extra trouble the treatment entails with the greatest zeal." He had authored a text on the handling of wounds antiseptically, which was translated into five languages and for which Lister "extended a personal affection."[27]

Lister's most magnificent reception came in Leipzig, where between three and four-hundred grateful admirers held a banquet and sang songs dedicated to him and his system. One of the melodies had been composed by university students and was given the title of "Carbolsäure Tingel-Tangel" or, as one historian has loosely translated it, "The Carbolic Acid Rag." Fifty or more of the students present had come from Halle with Professor Volkmann. The master of ceremonies was Karl Thiersch, the first surgeon to introduce the antiseptic method in Germany. Thiersch expressed a preference for salicylic acid over carbolic acid because the former was less toxic and irritating, which meant that it could be applied in higher concentrations and that wounds did not have to be dressed as often. It was not volatile and did not have a distinct odor, either. Lister felt duty-bound to defend carbolic acid, even though he was a guest. When the time came for him to speak, he rejected Thiersch's arguments. He did acknowledge salicylic acid's ability to keep dressings sweet but thought that it took too long to kill bacteria.[28]

One eyewitness account of Thiersch's opening remarks is especially good. Relating how the host had described Lister's accomplishments, the observer wrote,

---

[25] James G. Wakley, "High German Testimony to Antisepticism in Surgery," *The Lancet* (3 April 1875): 485–86.

[26] Fritz Linder and Hugh Forrest, "The Propagation of Lister's Ideas," *Surgery, Gynecology & Obstetrics* 132 (November 1968): 1083–84.

[27] Ibid; William Craig, "Medical News," *Edinburgh Medical Journal* 21 (July 1875): 92; James G. Wakley, "Professor Lister in Germany," *The Lancet* (19 June 1875): 868.

[28] Wakley, "Lister in Germany," p. 868; Richard B. Fisher, *Joseph Lister, 1827–1912* (New York: Stein and Day, 1977), p. 213; I. H. Upmalis, "The Introduction of Lister's Treatment in Germany," *Bulletin of the History of Medicine* 42 (May–June 1968): 232.

His discovery, like all other great ones, has had to pass through the usual three stages: the first, when the world smiles and shakes its head and says, "It's just nonsense;" the second, with a shrug of the shoulders, and a look of contempt, "It's the merest humbug;" and finally, "Oh, that's an old story; we knew that long ago." He next compared it to a foetus, which cannot develop itself in quiet and stillness, but, surrounded by meddling relations, the one saying, "This arm is too short," another, "This nose is too large," and a third, "This leg is too long,"—must grow up as best it can; yet, notwithstanding, owing to the skill and care of its father, it had grown up to be a strong, healthy, well-formed child, with whom everyone was satisfied.[29]

Coincidentally, shortly before Lister's tour of Germany, Thiersch had written an article on the successes he had experienced using the antiseptic technique during the period from April, 1874, to February, 1875. In it he referred to the Englishman's method of treating wounds as a "therapeutic experiment" that had to be tried "even if the scientific hypothesis is incomplete."[30]

Prior to leaving Germany Lister went to Halle, where he was entertained by Professor Volkmann, and then traveled to the nation's capital. There, he set aside one day for sightseeing and another for touring "the two important Berlin hospitals." He also enjoyed a private meal with one ,of Berlin's leading surgeons, A. Bardeleben.[31] Bardeleben was employed at Charite Hospital and was one of the earliest supporters of Lister's principle in Germany. In January, 1870, he had reported success with the antiseptic technique to the Medical Society of Berlin and had encouraged others to practice it. Two years later one of his assistants had journeyed to Edinburgh to study Lister's system; after returning to Berlin he published his findings, marking "the turning point in the history of antiseptic surgery in Germany."[32]

Lister seldom turned down an invitation to exhibit his technique, and once he was back in the British Isles, he applied it to ever more lengthy and complicated operations. On the fourth and fifth of August, 1875, he demonstrated his method to the members of the British Medical Association in the operating theater of the Edinburgh Royal Infirmary. (See Figure 14.) The first day of the conference he performed surgery on a patient's knee-joint, which was kept open with a drainage tube. To have left the incision exposed without the use of antiseptics would have been calamitous. By applying carbolic acid to the surrounding skin and providing for free discharge through India-rubber tubing, however, Lister was not only able to prevent inflammation but also relieved the pressure which results from the buildup of large amounts of fluid following procedures of that type. Healing was therefore expedited and greater mobility of the joint resulted. He later presented patients to the assembly who had undergone successful operations for injuries to anklebones, thighbones, and shinbones.[33]

---

[29] William Craig, "Correspondence," *Edinburgh Medical Journal* 21 (July 1875): 94.
[30] Upmalis, "Lister's Treatment in Germany," p. 231.
[31] Fisher, *Joseph Lister,* pp. 214–15.
[32] Upmalis, "Lister's Treatment in Germany," pp. 224–27.
[33] Joseph Lister, "Demonstrations of Antiseptic Surgery," *Edinburgh Medical Journal* 21 (September 1875): 193–94, 200, 203, 204.

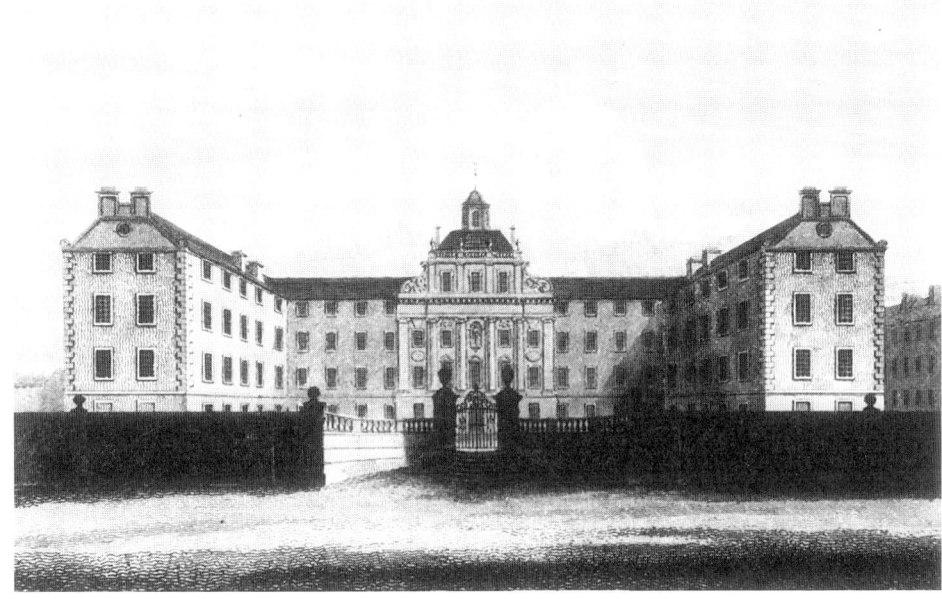

Figure 14. Edinburgh Royal Infirmary

During Lister's presentation to the British Medical Association, he constantly insisted on the crucial importance of the carbolic-acid spray for success in surgery, especially during operations involving body cavities. He even announced an improvement in the administration of carbolic acid atmospherically that must have seemed trivial to his listeners. Now, instead of setting the machine to dispense the antiseptic at a right angle, it was adjusted to provide spray at a forty-five degree incline. This meant that not as much spray landed on the surgeon's hands and arms, whereas before it had always soaked his coat sleeves. Lister described the mist that resulted as "little coarser than a London fog."

Clearly, Lister was trying to respond to surgeons who had rejected the spray because it was so disagreeable. He later confessed that if he "could dispense with the spray, no one would rejoice more than myself; but until somebody wiser than I am can supply some better means, we must continue to use it." Although he tried to make his technique less unpleasant and easier to implement, he believed that it would be "far better that the antiseptic method should not be employed at all than that it should be used imperfectly." He cited a surgeon who misdirected the spray as an example. Apparently forgetting what had happened to Queen Victoria, Lister concluded that "such attempts not only end in disappointment, but throw discredit on the system."[34] As correct as his appraisal of the situation was, Lister was partly at fault for the slow adoption of his technique because he expected so much of the medical profession that many surgeons refused to even try it. It required extreme devotion for surgeons and their assistants, who spent as much as two hours in major operations, to work with

---

[34] Ibid., pp. 195, 197–98.

spray machines, especially those powered by bellows instead of steam, and then to find themselves soaked with carbolic acid once the surgery was over.

On the second day of its meeting, the British Medical Association discussed another of Lister's favorite topics: antiseptically treated catgut ligatures. Again, he was characteristically arrogant in his summation of their worth. He preened, "I believe myself that this is a pretty perfect method of obstructing a vessel in its continuity; I do not see that we can wish to have it improved upon." In his defense, however, it must be noted that this time he attributed failures by others in the use of such ligatures to his own oversight in not meticulously describing the various stages of their preparation. Regardless of the mistake and who made it, whether it was spraying carbolic acid in the wrong direction or not steeping carbolized ligatures properly, the message that the members of the association got was that the antiseptic method was complicated from beginning to end. Oblivious to this fact Lister maintained that if his prescription was followed to the letter "there will be no further complaints about untrustworthiness of the catgut."[35]

Between the published accounts of Lister's two-day demonstration of surgical procedures, which were printed in the *Edinburgh Medical Journal* three months apart, an epic poem appeared. It was entitled "Antisepticism: a Fytte," and it highlighted the very aspects of Lister's practice that were described at the convention. The anonymous author used numerous puns to tell the story of the antiseptic system. He quipped that Lister was not blowing his own trumpet, but a cloud of carbolic acid spray instead, and that Lister vowed it would not go up in smoke like a cloud of tobacco. As he ended his jocular stanzas, the writer expressed his fear that he might "draw down a *dressing*" for his long-windedness, but not an antiseptic one.[36]

Regardless of the absurdity of the antiseptic method to some, careful surgeons who desired to perform dangerous and complex operations gradually began to try Lister's technique and to attest to the advances made possible by it.[37] Knee surgery was traditionally very dangerous, and one of its main practitioners was Thomas Pickering Pick, a surgeon at the Belgrave Hospital for Children in London. In an address to the London Clinical Society, he stated that he had not had a single instance of unhealthy discharge, erysipelas, or pyemia since adopting the use of carbolic acid. One of his patients had died from the last of these scourges, but it was an individual who had not been treated antiseptically. In spite of his support for Lister, Pick was typical of many surgeons who did not really comprehend the principle underlying the technique. He did not think that carbolic acid "prevented suppuration nor that it hastened union, but that it prevented the *decomposition* of pus, which was what we had to dread."[38]

Another surgeon in London, Timothy Holmes, told the society that he had complete confidence in the ability of carbolic acid to stop suppuration. He rejected the germ theory, however, and downplayed the perception that hospital deaths from pyemia were prevalent. He did this by producing post-mortem statistics from his place

---

[35] Ibid., (December 1875): 481–83.

[36] *Seria mista jocis* [pseud.], "Antisepticism: a Fytte," *Edinburgh Medical Journal* 21 (October 1875): 377, 382.

[37] James G. Wakley, "Clinical Society of London," *The Lancet* (16 October 1875): 562.

[38] Ibid., (30 October 1875): 628.

of employment, St. George's Hospital. Publishing the numbers for three separate years, he showed that the proportion of deaths from the disease was actually quite low when compared to the overall mortality figures. For example, of two-hundred and forty-one deaths the preceding year only eleven were attributable to pyemia. It is possible that these computations accurately portray the extent to which pyemia contributed to fatalities at St. George's Hospital; indeed, another study conducted a century later seems to substantiate Holmes's premise. It is also evident, though, that the managers of the institution had simply been unable to assess properly which deaths were specifically due to infectious bacteria.[39]

In addition to objections to the theory on which his method was based and to his claim that it prevented suppuration, others took issue with technical aspects of Lister's procedure. Predictably, one of the most heated debates concerned the practicality of the spray. Christopher Heath of University College Hospital, who had personally toured Lister's wards in Edinburgh just prior to attending the most recent meeting of the British Medical Association there, referred to the spray as "repellent" and noted that "he had almost resolved each time he employed it not to do it again." More judicious in his handling of the difficulties associated with antiseptic operations was Thomas Smith of St. Bartholomew's Hospital who exhorted his fellow surgeons to stop dissecting Lister's system and agree to either "accept his method *in toto* or reject it altogether." The most astute observation came from Richard Barwell of Charing Cross Hospital, who reasoned that surgeons would not endeavor to implement Lister's technique, no matter how beneficial it was, if they found the "details" to be "repulsive." He also responded defensively to Smith's admonition and called for a simplification of the antiseptic technique. In Barwell's opinion, Lister had hurt himself by developing a system that was so "mixed up."[40]

Wakley agreed with Barwell that Lister had done his own cause harm. He described Lister's method with the adjectives "extremely complicated, expensive, irksome, and laborious" and reported in late 1875 that there was "less antiseptic surgery practised in the metropolitan hospitals than ever there was." He then referred to the time that had passed since the first operation based on the antiseptic principle had been performed:

> It has been very pertinently remarked that if the special merits of Mr. Lister's plan were really as great as they are alleged to be, they should at the expiration of eight or ten years have declared themselves with overwhelming force and certainty. If the antiseptic system were really all that it is claimed to be, not the shadow of a doubt of its immense superiority over every other system should now exist. But the reverse is the case.[41]

Wakley then alluded to an unnamed hospital in London where one practitioner "strictly and exclusively" adhered to Lister's system while all others in the institution

[39] Ibid; John Woodward, *To do the sick no harm: A study of the British voluntary hospital system to 1875* (London: Routledge & Kegan Paul, 1974), p. 166.
[40] Wakley, "Clinical Society," (30 October 1875): 628–29; F. F. Cartwright, "Antiseptic Surgery," in *Medicine and Science in the 1860s*, ed. F. N. L. Poynter (London: Wellcome Institute for the History of Medicine, 1968), p. 98.
[41] James G. Wakley, "Antiseptic Surgery," *The Lancet* (16 October 1875): 565.

refused to give it a trial. When the results obtained from the two opposing strategies were compared, the antiseptic technique fared no better than ordinary methods and was "stated to be actually less" effective over a period of years.[42] Wakley's explanation for the decline in mortality, especially in Continental hospitals, was that the institutions themselves had been improved subsequent to James Y. Simpson's warnings concerning "hospitalism." He even went so far as to label the praises of European surgeons for the antiseptic system "extravagant," minimizing the significance of their testimony as "not therefore of much special value." It was ironic that Wakley should credit Simpson, Lister's most outspoken adversary, with the advances that Lister's technique had made in surgery.[43]

Another obvious paradox in the renewed debate over the antiseptic system in London was that Lister's foes seemed to put "unlimited faith" in his carbolized catgut ligatures, but remained skeptical of his principle in general. Wakley, himself, admitted that they could be accused of giving credence to the very method they regarded as incredible by supporting "a minute quantity" of carbolic acid while at the same time opposing its "free use." Yet, he justified this inconsistency by rationalizing that the ligatures prepared with carbolic acid were not antiseptic in the strictest sense, unless they were covered with antiseptic dressings after being tied, because they lost their disinfectant a short time later. He conveniently ignored what happened to the substance after it left the sutures.[44]

Even antiseptic dressings caused controversy, especially at the Clinical Society of London. At one of its meetings in late 1875, Marcus Beck, a surgeon at University College Hospital and Lister's brother-in-law, felt compelled to issue what Wakley termed "the formal protest of an advocate." Beck emphatically declared that the antiseptic method of dressing wounds was being "systematically neglected." He found this tragic because Lister "had always held and stated that in a few hours after the ligature there was no trace of carbolic acid left in the wound." This meant that without the addition of an antiseptic dressing, there was nothing to stop the occurrence of suppuration. Wakley did not share Beck's concern and counted "but few of the speakers" at the society's sessions who accepted the germ theory or embraced all of the facets of the antiseptic technique. He then elaborated on this broad generalization by adding an exaggeration: "It would be difficult to name more than one or two who are thoroughgoing believers in the theory, and there are scarcely more who strictly and fully carry out the practice."[45]

Had he looked more closely, Wakley would have found a third surgeon to add to his list of Lister's supporters. N. Davies-Colley of Guy's Hospital submitted two articles for the official publication of his institution, in which he enthusiastically wrote that the antiseptic method of wound management "bids fair to supersede all other plans of operative treatment" for "the radical cure of varicose veins in the lower extremity." He had been emboldened to try the complicated procedure after witnessing "with what safety the synovial cavities of joints and the sheaths of tendons might be

[42] Ibid.
[43] Ibid., (23 October 1875): 597–98.
[44] James G. Wakley, "The Debate on Antiseptic Surgery," *The Lancet* (20 November 1875): 743.
[45] Ibid; Wakley, "Clinical Society," (20 November 1875): 738; Cartwright, "Antiseptic Surgery," p. 98.

opened" using carbolic acid, "without fear of exciting suppuration or diffuse inflammation."[46] Success with that endeavor led Davies-Colley to attempt resecting a patient's shoulder-joint according to Lister's principle. Again, he enjoyed what he described as a "fortunate result," and there was no impairment of mobility in the limb.
His good fortune, he said, was "much aided by the use of the antiseptic treatment,"
which he clearly stressed "was carefully followed out."[47]

As 1875 ended it became apparent that Lister's system was being vigorously discussed by members of the London medical profession. It was equally plain to see that
regardless of his reception on the Continent, Lister would have to convince those in
England's capital of the value of his method by demonstrating it in their presence.
Only then would they be persuaded to either accept his principle or remain true to
tradition. Before he was given an opportunity to move to London, though, his lieuten-
ants in Scotland and Ireland took up the campaign for the antiseptic technique in one
last effort to win over Lister's critics.

In January, 1876, Wakley published an article by Cameron entitled "Illustrations
of Antiseptic Surgery." A surgeon at the Glasgow Royal Infirmary, Cameron described
his experience with cases of open knee-joint surgery in order to outline the clinical
features of the antiseptic technique. He also expressed consternation toward those who
persisted in deprecating Lister's system by citing cases where patients were cured with
other plans. The issue was not whether the antiseptic principle was the only approach
that would work in all instances, Cameron argued, but what the safest method and
the one most likely to succeed was. Nevertheless, while admitting the possibility of
success without employing Lister's procedure, Cameron distinguished between it and
the other modes of treatment; if they failed to unite the wound by "first intention,"
suppuration was unavoidable, but if the antiseptic system faltered in bringing about
closure, the surgical incision or injured opening would still be free from putrefaction.[48]

A. J. Youngson has elaborated on the significance of healing by first intention, as
opposed to second intention, in his study of Victorian medicine. He describes first
intention healing as coming about "without inflammation or suppuration." Second
intention healing came about "through the gradual filling of the cavity with a rudi-
mentary form of tissue called granulations, the process being a prolonged one, accompanied by more or less inflammation and suppuration and probably fever." "Until
Lister had done his work," writes Youngson,

> healing by first intention was scarcely expected, save after operations on certain
> parts of the body, such as the face. Healing by second intention was the rule. In
> this latter case, if all went well, post-operational suppuration, inflammation and
> fever were not prolonged. The flow of pus from the openings provided for drain-
> age gradually diminished after the first week or two, the wound became less in-
> flamed, the fever subsided, and after several weeks or even months, the patient

---

[46] N. Davies-Colley, "Two Cases of Varicose Veins of the Lower Extremity Treated by Excision," *Guy's Hospital Reports,*
Third Series, 20 (1875): 431.
[47] N. Davies-Colley, "Case of Partial Resection of the Head of the Humerus," *Guy's Hospital Reports,* Third Series, 20
(1875): 525, 529.
[48] Hector C. Cameron, "Illustrations of Antiseptic Surgery," *The Lancet* (22 January 1876): 123–24.

recovered. Surgeons were well satisfied with such a result, 'and were full of self-congratulations if anything better was achieved'.[49]

Youngson's quote came from Rickman Godlee, Lister's nephew, who understood that something better could be achieved with the antiseptic method. This was precisely the same point Cameron made in his illustrative essay. Cameron encouraged his readers to use Lister's method because of "how monotonous generally is the daily record of a successful antiseptic case." Cameron emphasized that there was little or no follow-up to such cases, which contradicted the charge some had made that Lister's approach involved more time, effort, and material than other systems. Cameron had found, relevant to these three factors, that in situations where wounds did not become putrid the antiseptic technique was so predictable that it was "economical in respect of all of them." Moving from the sublime to the ridiculous to make his point about the predictability of Lister's system, he included the account of a weakly, old patient who expired from factors unrelated to her wound, but whose surgical site revealed that her injury had been successfully treated and was healing nicely.[50] Clearly, although all else had failed, the antiseptic system worked.

Perhaps inspired by Cameron's initial onslaught, others began coming forward to fight for Lister and the triumph of his system over the professional envy, philosophical bias, and national conceit that existed in London. From Ireland came a notice substantiating Cameron's assertion that an antiseptic operation could be performed in the same amount of time and with no greater difficulty than other kinds of surgery. The one who informed surgeons in the Emerald Isle of these facts anticipated some objections to the intricacies of Lister's technique and deflected them by conveying "that attention to these details appears much more troublesome in description than they are in practice." He also summarized a victory he had won by following them, the removal of lower knee-joint cartilage. He deduced that "the antiseptic mode of dressing . . . aided materially in procuring the almost complete immunity from inflammation which the patient enjoyed, and which rendered this hazardous operation successful."[51]

In the spring and summer of 1876, two clinical lectures on the antiseptic method appeared in *The Lancet*. They were delivered by Thomas Smith of London's St. Bartholomew's Hospital as part of a one-year investigation of Lister's system. He applied the antiseptic principle to "test cases," which he explained were those "cases where the antiseptic method is fairly put on its trial, and where an opportunity occurs for such advantages as it is said to possess to become plainly apparent." These cases included resections of large joints, compound fractures, and deep or chronic abscesses. Smith also agreed to the "two preliminary conditions" set forth by Lister for anyone who undertook to prove or disprove the truth of antiseptic surgery. They were "that they should at least provisionally accept his theory" and "that they should know what his practice is, and should carry it out even to the minutest particular." Smith had met

[49] A. J. Youngson, *The Scientific Revolution in Victorian Medicine* (New York: Holmes & Meier Publishers, Inc., 1979), p. 32.
[50] Cameron, "Illustrations," (22 January 1876): 124; (29 January 1876): 166, 168.
[51] John K. Barton, "Two Cases Illustrating the Advantages of the Antiseptic Treatment of Wounds," *The Dublin Journal of Medical Science* 61 (March 1876): 229, 234.

the latter requirement by personally visiting Edinburgh to learn Lister's practice, and in regard to the former stipulation, he merely reoriented his thinking to concur with the germ theory "for the present at least."[52]

The last paragraph of his first speech indicated which way Smith was leaning in his inquiry. He simply asked his readers to equate experimentation in medicine with comparable research in other disciplines and to have as much patience for those who deal with organic matter as for those who work with inorganic substances. He reminded them of the studies of John Tyndall, and asked his readers

> to observe that even in the chemical laboratory there are difficulties to be overcome and minute details to be observed in order to obtain uniform results; and that, even in the hands of masters of the art, notwithstanding all care, sources of error will sometimes occur, and a fallacious result be obtained. Now, if this be the case under the circumstances I have referred to, how much more difficult must it be to carry out the necessary details when beginners like ourselves are dealing with the living tissues of the human body.[53]

It was also important, he pointed out, for surgeons to appreciate the limitations of antisepsis and not to condemn Lister's method when it was ineffective in the treatment of contaminated wounds. They had to understand that "Lister does not claim a certainty of success in the antiseptic treatment of operation wounds, unless he has to deal with the unbroken skin."[54]

Lister, however, was not known for readily admitting that his system was less than perfect. The numerous changes he made in it attested to its imperfection, but his stubborn insistence that it be adopted in every minute detail sounded very much like he thought that it was the only method that could conscientiously be employed. English surgeons were just as obstinate and felt just as superior, particularly in London, and before they were willing to believe, they had to see with their own eyes. In the meantime Lister received exaltation in the eyes of the Germans and took his doctrine to the United States. Only when his fame and exposure grew elsewhere, did his native country reconsider its rejection of him, finally honoring him with the opportunity to spread his gospel at home.

---

[52] Thomas Smith, "Clinical Lectures on Lister's Treatment of Wounds and Abscesses by the Antiseptic Method," *The Lancet* (25 March 1876): 453.

[53] Ibid., p. 455.

[54] Ibid., (1 July 1876): 5.

8. Surgical Demonstration as a Factor in the Diffusion of Listerism

By August of 1876 it was clear that a sizable dent had been made in the defenses of Lister's London opponents. Even Wakley could not ignore the impact of Thomas Smith and others. A careful reading of the editor's words betrays a noticeable change in strategy from attacking antisepticism to trying tenaciously to ensure that traditional measures remained part of surgical technique. After printing that Lister's practice was "obtaining increasing attention," Wakley hastily pointed out that "it cannot be said that it is as yet universally adopted." He then unknowingly reflected the isolation of those in London who still resisted the antiseptic principle by adding, "At least, judging from London, it is found that in some hospitals faith is weaker than in others, and there are certain groups of surgeons who adhere to the old system."[1]

Wakley obviously still preferred the open-air form of wound treatment, but to defend it he disgraced himself; he tried to impugn Lister's popularity by reporting that the French were "very lukewarm" when it came to the antiseptic method. Wakley did admit that the Germans had subscribed to it "with enthusiasm," and he grudgingly noted "that much has been gained within the last few years." Yet, throughout his editorials an air of stubbornness and condescension was unmistakable. He was right about France because Lister's technique had only been adopted by a few surgeons there. The leading French proponent of the antiseptic system was Just Lucas-Championniere of Paris, who had visited Lister's wards in Glasgow in 1868 but had not attempted a "rigorously precise application" of his principle until 1875. He had to pay for all the materials necessary to carry out the method himself, and many of his associates were not receptive. However, by the following year he had made converts and had "prevailed upon the administration of the hospitals to furnish the materials for the dressing."[2]

Although Lister was clearly gaining adherents in Europe, enthusiasm for his method had not traveled across the Atlantic. He went to America in September, 1876, for the centennial of the independence of the United States. He had been asked to attend the International Medical Congress, which was held in Philadelphia as part of the anniversary celebration, and he was appointed chairman of the surgical section. Lister was personally well received, and at the banquet which followed sat by President Grant, but he was unable to convince his skeptical American audience of the efficacy of his system.

This skepticism was due in part to the stature of Samuel Gross, the president of the convention and the author of the most widely used American textbook on surgery. Gross was a leading opponent of Lister and had been the subject of a painting the year before that depicted his blatant contempt for all things antiseptic. Thomas Eakins's

---

[1] James G. Wakley, "The Antiseptic Methods," *The Lancet* (19 August 1876): 267–68.
[2] Ibid; Just Lucas-Championniere, *Antiseptic Surgery: The Principles, Modes of Application, and Results of the Lister Dressing* (Portland, Maine: Loring, Short, and Harmon, 1881), pp. 9–10.

famous canvas was fittingly titled "The Gross Clinic." Gross's views were shared by most of the four-hundred and eighty participants at the medical conference. The American Medical Association refused to sanction the antiseptic method, and Lister's tour was hardly mentioned in the medical papers of the United States.[3] One periodical that did publish a synopsis of Lister's Philadelphia address was the *Boston Medical and Surgical Journal.* In portraying him it read, "Modesty is stamped upon his every act and word, but he *does* believe in antiseptic surgery." It also reported that he said a new era had dawned in performing operations. Gross reacted by saying that "irritative fever" had been prevented in his patients for years without using Lister's method.[4]

By the end of 1876 Wakley and other dogmatic opponents of Lister's principle were becoming increasingly isolated as knowledge of the system spread beyond Europe's medical capitals. As a country practitioner in Scotland phrased it, "The splendid results obtained through the practice of antiseptic surgery cannot but have excited in every one, liable to be called on to perform an operation, the desire to avail himself of the improvement."[5] More and more, surgeons were adopting Lister's technique, ignoring the philosophical arguments over Pasteur's theory, rejecting the power of the medical press, and relinquishing their own time-honored traditions. Lister himself had perceived the change that was taking place in the attitude of the medical profession. Before leaving for America he had urged the graduating class at the University of Edinburgh to think independently, to search for truth regardless of whether it was popular or not, and to be honest, "considering that the weakness of our nature makes it often hard for men to recant an error to which they have once committed themselves."[6] The ulterior motives of those who sustained their resistance to antiseptic surgery were rapidly becoming transparent and indefensible.

As faith in antiseptic surgery spread, the scent of carbolic acid began to become part of every conceivable kind of surgical intervention. For example, Edward Bennett, a professor of surgery at the University of Dublin, adopted Lister's method for the treatment of empyema, the accumulation of pus in the pleural cavity. Instead of injecting antiseptics into the cavity, as was commonly done, he made a free incision and allowed the fluids to drain. The most important advantages of this new way of dealing with the sickness were that decomposition and absorption of pus were prevented, the lining of the thorax was not irritated, and the process did not have to be repeated as often.[7]

Indeed, the fervor of Lister's disciples often verged on the hysterical, and their enthusiasm reached a peak in 1877 when he was offered a position at King's College Hospital in London. The cause for the climax was Lister's response to a petition from more than seven hundred of his students asking him to stay in Edinburgh. The students wrote of Lister's "self-devotion" and "indomitable energy" and described his in-

---

[3] Richard B. Fisher, *Joseph Lister, 1827–1912* (New York: Stein and Day, 1977), pp. 223–24; Sherwin B. Nuland, *Doctors: The Biography of Medicine* (New York: Alfred A. Knopf, 1988), p. 372.
[4] Quoted in Nuland, *Doctors,* p. 372; William Craig, "Periscope," *Edinburgh Medical Journal* 22 (November 1876): 464, 466.
[5] John Balfour, "Antiseptic for Country Practice," *Edinburgh Medical Journal* 22 (August 1876): 103.
[6] William Craig, "Medical News," *Edinburgh Medical Journal* 22 (September 1876): 280–84.
[7] Edward H. Bennett, "A Case of Empyema, Complicated by Pleural Fistula, Treated Successfully by the Antiseptic Method of Lister," *The Dublin Journal of Medical Science* 62 (November 1876): 361–62, 368.

fluence on them as "impossible to overrate." They also linked the well-being of their university to Lister's presence and stated that his departure would "be an irreparable loss." His response indicated that he would not accept the post, giving as his reasons that he could not deliver clinical lectures in surgery or take his assistants with him. The concluding sentence of the signed plea for his continued presence in Scotland, however, contained the words, "We are far from disparaging that field to which you may be called."[8]

To Wakley, this kind of enthusiasm went beyond the bounds of propriety or good sense, and in a vitriolic editorial he not only reproved Lister in the strongest possible terms but also insinuated that the pupils protested too much to be taken seriously. "To be pronounced the founder of a system of surgery," it read,

> is certainly apt to make a man feel proud, but to be told that his example has given "a mental impetus for good, the effects of which it is impossible to over-rate," may be allowed to be sufficient to engender a spark of vanity in the humblest breast. At least Mr. Lister has shown that he is not proof against the seductions of this form of flattery. After receiving the complimentary memorial of his pupils last week, he seems to have lost himself in infatuation, and, without questioning the truth or value of the sentiments of his memorialists, so far forgot are the rules of decency and good taste as to contemptuously decline an offer that had never been made to him. But his elation would not suffer him to stop even there, for, like a man who in the excitement of enthusiasm raves at the false creations of his heat-oppressed brain, Mr. Lister fancied he saw in his professional *confrères* in London only unsubstantial shades and showy shams. After contrasting what he ungraciously designated the gropings of physicians with his own demonstrations "in the actual living flesh and blood" of his patients, he proceeded to stigmatise the teaching of clinical surgery in London, compared with the method which he employs, as "a mere sham."[9]

Lister had actually been approached informally about the chair in clinical surgery that had been left vacant by the death of William Fergusson. However, it was ultimately given to John Wood, who was next in seniority and reportedly opposed hiring Lister. Lister told his brother that he had received a letter from William Overend Priestley of King's College Hospital which indicated "that Mr. Wood made such strong objections to the idea of an outsider being appointed over his head, declaring that he would leave King's altogether if it occurred, that it was concluded that it would be out of the question to ask me to go there."[10]

Convinced that his best opportunity to go to London had "fallen through," Lister resigned himself to staying in Edinburgh and pensively informed the editor of *The British Medical Journal* of his decision: "So myself personally I have felt the scales

[8] G. T. Wrench, *Lord Lister: His Life and Work* (New York: Frederick A. Stokes Company, 1914), pp. 267–70.
[9] James G. Wakley, "Professor Lister," *The Lancet* (10 March 1877): 361.
[10] Joseph Lister to Arthur Lister, 27 February 1877, Western Manuscripts, Wellcome Institute for the History of Medicine, London, MS 6968, 6; Fisher, *Joseph Lister,* pp. 224–25, 229; F. F. Cartwright, "Lister—The Man," *The British Journal of Surgery* 54 (Supplement 1967): 408.

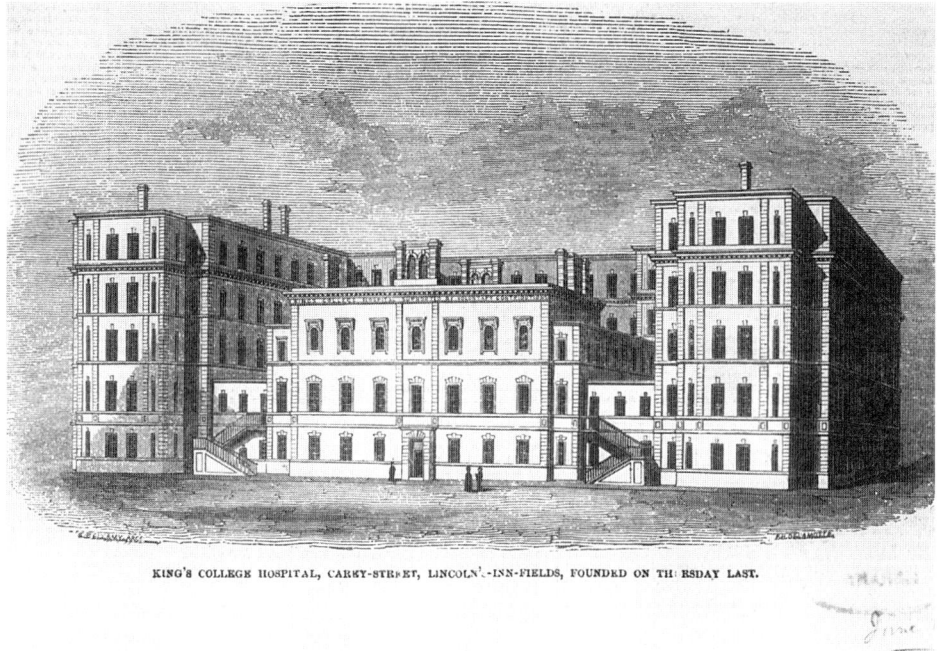

KING'S COLLEGE HOSPITAL, CAREY-STREET, LINCOLN'.-INN-FIELDS, FOUNDED ON TH RSDAY LAST.

Figure 15. King's College Hospital

weighted so evenly that I find it easy to fall back into the belief that my position here is that in which I can best serve my generation." Many members of the King's College Hospital Board, however, feared that the publicity caused by the controversy would negatively impact their institution, and they needed more medical students. Consequently, they voted to create a second chair in clinical surgery, reopened one ward that had not been used for years, built another one, and formally offered Lister a position consistent with his stipulations.[11] (See Figure 15.)

Lister's last lecture in Edinburgh was at the end of July, 1877, and two months later he returned to his own country where so many had refused to honor him. Between the time when he was first contacted by its administrators and when he was hired by King's College Hospital, surgeons in London did not hesitate to comment on Lister's stated opinion of them. Thomas Bryant of Guy's Hospital, for example, defended his institution and argued that it was "not contemptible," whether or not it was "the best in theory." He felt that, in practice, they had a good system and added that "if their opportunities have been neglected to a great extent, it is because the material with which they have been supplied has been so profuse that it has not been within their power to turn it all to a demonstrative account."[12] In other words, Bryant believed that there were too many patients in London's hospitals for the antiseptic

[11] Joseph Lister to Ernest Hart, 28 March 1877, Western Manuscripts, Wellcome Institute for the History of Medicine, London, MS 5424, 8; Fisher, *Joseph Lister,* pp. 230–31.
[12] Thomas Bryant, "Professor Lister and Clinical Surgery in the London Hospitals," *The Lancet* (10 March 1877): 367–68.

system to be implemented effectively. It was precisely the opportunity to change the theoretical base of London medical practice, and to prove that his principle could be applied in the larger metropolitan hospitals, that inspired Lister to accept the challenge of going to England's capital.

Bryant had personally employed Lister's method for the first time eight years earlier, and his results had normally been successful. Then, he had ascribed his effectiveness to carbolic acid, but in *Guy's Hospital Reports* for 1877 he was very cautious in recommending the substance because he had found "great nervous depression and semi-unconsciousness to be a direct consequence of its use." H. G. Howse, a fellow surgeon at Guy's Hospital, took exception to his colleague's observations and noted that in a seven-year period he had "not had a single case . . . of poisoning by carbolic acid." Bryant's problems apparently stemmed from his use of carbolic acid in solutions that were four times as powerful as those used by Howse. Throughout the period of controversy, such abuses of Lister's technique ultimately explained many of its failures, particularly in London.[13]

Even though Bryant did not follow the antiseptic plan exactly as prescribed by Lister, Thomas Smith did and was quick to call upon Lister to retract the "hard words" that had been spoken against the London medical establishment. Smith, who had helped prepare the way for Lister's move to the metropolis with his year-long study of the antiseptic system, assured his colleagues that Lister did not view clinical instruction there as "a mere sham." He did agree that Lister had "an indifferent opinion" of the system ordinarily practiced in London, but that "the circumstances of the case scarcely warrant" the words he chose to describe it.[14] Lister took Smith's advice and three weeks later published an explanation of what he really meant. He supplied a long excerpt from his response to the students' petition which put his remarks in context.

Lister admitted that he did use the words "a mere sham" to characterize the "*system of the London Chairs of Clinical Surgery*" but claimed that he "was alluding to clinical surgery as taught in lectures, and not at all to clinical surgical instruction conducted otherwise." He attributed the misunderstanding of his comments to the fact that the Chair of Clinical Surgery at Edinburgh was like no other in the British Isles. Twice a week the professor lectured to his pupils in an operating theater where demonstrations could be made, and whoever was appointed to the position was considered equal to a teacher of systematic surgery. Other schools simply gave instruction at the bedside, to far fewer students at a time and in a fashion that was "essentially fragmentary in character, dealing in the main with isolated practical details." Also, professors in England taught both systematic and clinical surgery whereas the disciplines were kept distinct in Scotland. Wakley naturally saw Lister's attempt to clarify what he had said as an effort to justify himself. Lister's defense, wrote Wakley, "besides being one-sided and inconsistent, is wholly irrelevant."[15]

Lister moved to London on September 11, 1877, and began teaching on the first day of October. The hospital's administration made it mandatory for the students to

[13] H. G. Howse, "On the Use of Carbolic Acid in Surgical Dressings," *Guy's Hospital Reports*, Third Series, 22 (1877): 506–507.

[14] Thomas Smith, "Professor Lister and Clinical Surgery in the London Hospitals," *The Lancet* (10 March 1877): 368.

[15] Joseph Lister, "Clinical Surgery in London and Edinburgh," *The Lancet* (31 March 1877): 475–77.

attend his classes, though "the mere handful" of them could not compare to the four hundred he taught in Edinburgh. His conditions had been met, but he was only given twenty-four beds, far fewer than the sixty to which he was accustomed. The administrators even allowed him to bring his assistants with him.[16] Neither Lister nor his four Scottish helpers were well received at first. During his initial lecture, the medical students in attendance "heckled and stamped so that he could hardly be heard." The hospital's nurses objected when Lister and his assistants wanted to dress their patient's wounds.

Indeed, the attitudes of students, nurses, and co-workers were so hostile that one historian suspects they "would not have been possible if they had not been indoctrinated by their seniors with a spirit of antagonism towards this invader from the north."[17] Even a patient, who had been under Lister's care in Edinburgh, journeyed south to find her entrance into King's College Hospital blocked by one of the staff members because she did not have the proper papers to be admitted. This was all the more inexcusable because a basket, used to move patients from their hospital beds to the operating table, had been converted into a permanently suspended berth so that she could make the trip to London by train.[18]

The British Medical Journal announced Lister's arrival with a front page article that said he would contribute "to the glory and greatness of the surgical profession in London." Wakley ignored his arrival, though, which was interesting since he had been one of the leading backers of Lister in his bid for the chair in Edinburgh eight years before.[19] *The Lancet* did carry a brief summary of Lister's inaugural address at King's College, simply noting that he spoke on the fermentation of milk and described putrefaction as a process caused by the fermentation of the blood. Lister had ventured to prove to his listeners that all true fermentative processes were due to the action of microorganisms.[20] One person in the audience, St. Clair Thomson, who later became Lister's house-surgeon, wrote that with every reference to cows by Lister the students "tried to emit the 'Boo' of that animal; each time that he mentioned the contaminating hand of the dairy-maid we said 'tut-tut.'"[21]

As 1877 drew to a close, Timothy Holmes, the surgeon in London who did not believe the germ theory but did hold that carbolic acid prevented suppuration, submitted an article to Wakley's journal suggesting that the following year would be an ideal time to compare the success of Lister with that of Wood. Since Wood had abandoned the use of antiseptics on a regular basis, Holmes called on him to practice conventional methods of healing until the results could be analyzed. The "ordinary cases" were the ones Holmes wanted studied instead of "exceptional operations."[22]

Holmes was alluding to surgeries like those on the knee joint, which Lister had performed to the astonishment of two-hundred medical students and surgeons at

---

[16] Archibald Malloch, "Biographical Sketch and Memorabilia of Lister," *Supplement to the Bulletin of the New York Academy of Medicine* 4 (January 1928): 145; Fisher, *Joseph Lister,* pp. 230–31, 233.
[17] Jack Penn, "Lord Lister," *Medical Proceedings* 11 (3 July 1965): 299.
[18] W. B. Howie and S. A. B. Black, "Sidelights on Lister: A Patient's Account of Lister's Care," *Journal of the History of Medicine and Allied Sciences* 32 (July 1977): 250.
[19] Quoted in Wrench, *Lord Lister,* p. 273.
[20] James G. Wakley, "King's College," *The Lancet* (6 October 1877): 488–89.
[21] Quoted in Fisher, *Joseph Lister,* p. 236.
[22] T. Holmes, "Antiseptic Surgery," *The Lancet* (15 December 1877): 900–901.

King's College the day before Holmes corresponded with Wakley. They were amazed because Lister had successfully operated on a patient whose condition was not life threatening. Surgeons considered this unethical before they learned the antiseptic technique, but Lister knew that it would show his complete confidence in his system. The broken kneecap was wired together and not only was the leg spared, as it would have been without surgery, but also there was complete recovery. Lister's method of healing fractured patellas brought him renown. As one writer has expressed the awe of those who witnessed the procedure, "the surgeons who came to scoff, stayed to learn."[23]

Lister published a lecture on the opening of the knee joint in *The Lancet* on January 5, 1878, and it included certain remarks on the teaching of clinical surgery. He began by telling those in attendance that he could point out a patient's ills in an operating room "very much better than by taking you to her bed in the ward." His regular class now numbered fifty, but he noted that on an earlier occasion he had taken fewer than half of them to the ward where they still had to line up "in two rows, so as to form an alley to admit the light from the window." In spite of that arrangement, they were still "in one another's way." Lister contrasted teaching in such a setting with the surgical arena in which he was performing, concluding that "only those who were very near the bed could see what would have been shown without any difficulty to the whole class at once in this place."[24]

Of more concern to Lister than the surgeon who taught at the bedside, though, was the physician who only inferred. The latter had "no opportunity of witnessing this healing process during life; and when he sees its effects on post-mortem examination, they are probably marred by the results of decomposition." This statement clarified what Lister had been talking about when he reacted to the petition of his Edinburgh students. He went on to explain that "medical diseases differ from surgical diseases not so much in their nature as in their situation; and the same great principles of pathology, and to a large extent of practice also, must guide alike the physician and the surgeon." Before ending his presentation, Lister finally apologized to the surgeons of London for having permitted "an expression to escape my lips which I should not have uttered under any circumstances had I supposed that my remarks were likely to be published."[25]

Timothy Holmes's proposal to chronicle the work of Lister and Wood had no sooner started than it was "abandoned" at Wood's request. He had just seen one of Lister's patients, who had a malignant limb amputated antiseptically two days earlier, "sitting up in bed and reading the paper, being free from pain and free from fever." The scene so profoundly affected him that he was "generous enough to disclaim any kind of rivalry, and invited Lister to teach him the antiseptic method."[26] (See Figure 16.) That the experiment was short-lived did not seem to matter to one reader of *The Lancet,* who looked upon it as a scientific rather than a surgical exercise. In his view

[23] Frederick F. Cartwright, *Joseph Lister: The Man Who Made Surgery Safe* (London: Weidenfeld & Nicolson, 1963), pp. 82–92; Penn, "Lord Lister," p. 299.
[24] Joseph Lister, "Clinical Lecture on a Case of Excision of the Knee-Joint, and on Horsehair as a Drain for Wounds; with Remarks on the Teaching of Clinical Surgery," *The Lancet* (5 January 1878): 5, 7–8.
[25] Ibid., p. 8.
[26] Wrench, *Lord Lister,* p. 279.

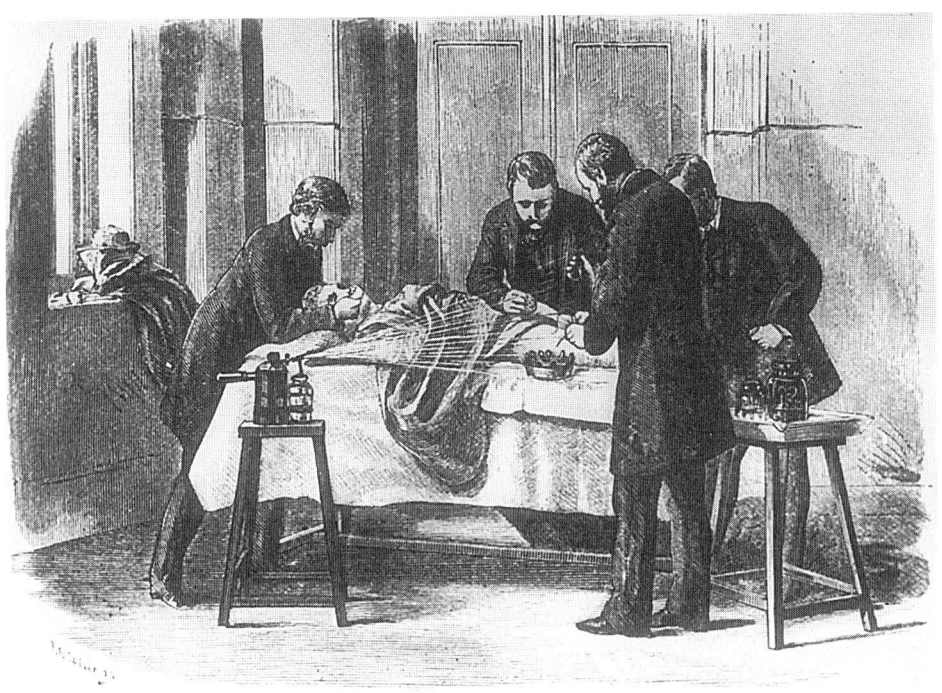

Figure 16. Antiseptic Surgery

the Germans had "eagerly adopted" Lister's practice because they were "scientific," and Scottish surgeons had incorporated it, "a little grudgingly," because they were "semi-scientific," but English surgeons had not embraced "the antiseptic doctrine" because they were "plodding and practical."[27]

To other English surgeons, who had tried Lister's technique over a period of one to three years, it did matter that the experiment proposed by Holmes ended so soon, and they started reporting their experiences. The longest discourse was that of Henry Davy, one of H. G. Howse's dressers, whose case histories of five patients were printed in the annual report of Guy's Hospital for 1878. They specifically dealt with the illness of pyemia, which had been deemphasized by Holmes as a leading cause of mortality in hospitals. Davy recorded that during the first six months of his employment as dresser for Howse, "hardly any rise" had been documented in the temperatures of his patients. He thought that it was due to his exercising "antiseptic precautions." It did not matter to him if germs induced putrefaction, only that carbolic acid and other chemicals forestalled the process. Moreover, antiseptics had been proven to deodorize the fluid which drained from wounds. He commended their use on that basis alone, regardless of their disinfecting action. He was much more interested in "the great practical point" of using antiseptics than "the theoretical reason" behind their use. Davy did comment on the fact that they got rid of injuries of "foreign matter," and, in his estimation, carbolic acid caused "all the discharges to percolate." He entreated others

[27] Flaneur [pseud.], "Antiseptic Surgery," *The Lancet* (5 January 1878): 36.

to apply Lister's system because he believed that it was the safest way to perform an operation.[28]

Many surgeons in England felt the same way about theory as Davy. Since numerous men, considered to be experts, had disagreed on a theory for explaining the cause of disease, the only reasonable thing to do was to achieve the best results possible. The debate over hospitalism, or nosocomial infections, had also apparently stopped in 1874. "The conclusion was, that Lister's insistence on cleanliness left nothing to be desired, whatever the theory might be." John Erichsen, the senior surgeon at University College Hospital, ventured to say that "practical surgery has nearly, if not quite, attained finality." In fact, he and most of the medical profession in England felt that the antiseptic system was unnecessarily protective, and "he saw no reason for going as far as Lister did."[29]

At about the same time that Davy's observations were made, Thomas Smith published the findings of his examination of Lister's method as part of the *St. Bartholomew's Hospital Reports*. His study, which was initially only supposed to last twelve months, took three years by the time he reported his results. He did not rely on "a statistical table" to validate his conclusions, but he did keep case histories of his patients. During the first year of the research, his house-surgeon had learned Lister's technique from the master himself and "was rewarded with commensurate success." However, the next two occupants of that post manifested "a certain laxity in the observance of antiseptic precautions, the result either of involuntary ignorance or invincible prejudice, and . . . this has been attended with a corresponding uncertainty of result."[30]

In every type of injury that Smith tested, Lister's method worked better than any of the other plans. Whether used to heal wounds to healthy joints, complications from diseased joints, compound fractures, or chronic abscesses, it was superior in that there was "very much less risk" and the "recovery seemed to be more complete." Not only was it a preferable mode of treatment but also, "under its aegis," Smith was able to "carry out to a successful issue operative measures, which . . . would be quite unjustifiable under other methods." Smith did find some problems with the antiseptic system: carbolic acid was extremely toxic to children, and secondary hemorrhages were difficult to detect beneath eight layers of gauze.[31]

Though Smith did not use statistics to verify the truth of his assertions, another surgeon in London did. The man who had taken exception to Smith's exhortation earlier, Richard Barwell, was now in agreement with his colleague that Lister had invented a system that was superior to any other. He produced a chart of thirty-five antiseptic surgeries, which revealed a mortality rate of only six percent, "from events unconnected with operation." This meant that "if death from extraneous causes be excluded," the number of his fatalities was "absolutely nil." He was so impressed by

---

[28] Henry Davy, "Five Cases Illustrative of Antiseptic Surgery and Pyaemia," *Guy's Hospital Reports*, Third Series, 23 (1878): 261, 264–65, 267–69.

[29] A. J. Youngson, *The Scientific Revolution in Victorian Medicine* (New York: Holmes & Meier Publishers, Inc., 1979), pp. 197–98.

[30] Thomas Smith, "Conclusions from a Personal Experience of Lister's Antiseptic Treatment during Three Years of Hospital Practice," *St. Bartholomew's Hospital Reports*, 14 (1878): 137–39.

[31] Ibid., pp. 139–44.

the "uniformly good result" he had achieved with "protected wounds" that he was convinced, in all cases handled antiseptically, similar success could "be reckoned upon with all but absolute certainty."[32]

Numerical data also came from a house-surgeon at the infirmary in Newcastle-on-Tyne. According to this surgeon, three years before the antiseptic technique was employed the death rate from amputations averaged fifty percent, as compared to twelve percent for the following three years. The one who furnished these figures concluded that they exhibited "the great security ensured by the adoption of Lister's method in large hospitals." Wakley, who published these statistics as well as those of Barwell, only said that a loss of half was "appalling, and whatever may be the representative value of 12 per cent for the antiseptic system, no one would pretend that 50 per cent is a fair average of the mortality under the best non-antiseptic methods."[33]

One month after Wakley begged the question about the proportional worth of Lister's practice, another infirmary surgeon described the successes he had in five minor operations using carbolic acid. His desire was to influence "those who have not yet found themselves able to believe that the antiseptic mode . . . must displace every other method yet brought forward, and that there is something more in it than careful drainage and absolute cleanliness." He acknowledged that, for a long time, he was "on the border-land of belief regarding the soundness of the doctrine on which it was based" but that he had been "driven" from his neutrality by what he "saw and heard" at Lister's wards in Edinburgh.[34]

In the last issue of *The Lancet* for 1878, a lecture by William Macewen was much more effective in swaying opinions than the slightly anecdotal cases mentioned earlier. He was the chest specialist at the Glasgow Royal Infirmary's clinic, and he must have stunned Lister's remaining critics when he stated, "I have now operated on over forty limbs and have performed over fifty osteotomies, without a single fatal case." He also had the distinction of being the first surgeon in Great Britain to execute an osteotomy, the removal or dividing of part of a bone, using antiseptics.[35] He had pioneered the procedure three years before, after learning of Lister's "intelligent treatment."

This onslaught stilled most English opponents of the antiseptic system, and the ever-critical Wakley had to rely on reports from other countries to portray antisepsis in an unfavorable light. He printed a correspondent's summary of a debate at the French Societe de Chirurgie on Lister's method of dressing wounds. Some in attendance resented the influx of "foreign innovations, which have invaded France several times this century, and always failed to effect the promised improvements." Others referred to Lister's "pretensions," pointing out that such breakthroughs as using carbolic acid in surgery, the advent of the drainage tube, the opening of chronic abscesses for antiseptic cleansing, and the employment of catgut ligature "belonged to the French school." According to them the one original contribution of Lister's practice "was the spray, and that had been shown to be useless." Actually, he was not the first

---

[32] Richard Barwell, "Some Statistics of Antiseptic Operations in the Year 1877," *The Lancet* (2 March 1878): 306–307.
[33] L. J. Hobson, "Antiseptic Surgery in Large Hospitals," *The Lancet* (8 June 1878): 851.
[34] J. C. Ogilvie Will, "Illustrations of Antiseptic Treatment in Minor Surgery," *The Lancet* (13 July 1878): 39; (20 July 1878): 79.
[35] Ibid., (13 July 1878): 39; William Macewen, "Lecture on Antiseptic Osteotomy for Genu Valgum, Genu Varum, and Other Osseous Deformities," *The Lancet* (28 December 1878): 911, 914.

to spray wounds with a carbolic acid solution; Thomas Nunn of Middlesex Hospital had achieved that distinction in 1868, but Lister was the one who began filling the atmosphere of operating theaters with the antiseptic.[36]

The way Lister's French antagonists defined original did not differentiate between successful attempts and failures, the most crucial consideration in determining claims of priority. They were correct about the impracticality of the carbolic-acid spray, though. Nearly everyone abandoned it before Lister did, with no ill effects. After reporting the general criticisms of Lister, Wakley's correspondent listed several specific items pertaining to the employment of antisepsis in France. News of osteotomies was looked upon with chagrin there because they were regarded as unnecessary in most cases, and Lister's technique had been found to be two percent less effective than other methods. Certain members of the French surgical society also stressed that Parisian surgeons, in particular, no longer subscribed to the antiseptic principle. However, the correspondent noted a very interesting omission on the part of Lister's detractors across the channel. They failed to record that the governmental agency regulating French hospitals discouraged any medical strategy that involved "expensive appliances." The reporter also questioned why the French would say that their ideas had been plagiarized if, as was claimed, those notions had not established a more beneficial system.[37]

When arguments against Lister's system were exposed as illogical, his opponents reverted to attacking the substance he had chosen as an antiseptic. It was a desperate act, but it had succeeded once before in persuading surgeons to avoid Lister's practice after it was first introduced. Once again articles started appearing which told of death from carbolic acid poisoning. Such scare tactics were so transparent this time that one surgeon's response defeated them and indicated the extent to which Lister's followers had been converted to his principle and the theory on which it was founded. James Grey Glover declared that "the antiseptic system applied to surgery is too marvellous in its results for even a general practitioner to be indifferent to any unfounded suggestion which might retard its general adoption."[38] He was replying to a fellow Londoner, A. Pearce Gould, who had implied that thrombosis in one of his cases of hip-joint surgery was the result of carbolic acid being absorbed into the blood. Even Gould acknowledged, though, "that the fortunes of antiseptic surgery are not bound up with those of carbolic acid."[39]

That was one of the lessons Lister had wanted the members of the medical profession to learn twelve years earlier, and he repeated it in Ireland in June, 1879. He went there to receive an honorary degree from the University of Dublin, and while he was there he told surgeons at Richmond Hospital, "I am not bound to any particular agent." He also stated that "the truth of the germ theory of putrefaction" should be taken "for granted." "Every year that passes," he said, "adds facts in favour of that theory, and tends to clear away any difficulties that may have been raised regarding

[36] James G. Wakley, "Paris," *The Lancet* (19 April 1879): 574–75; James G. Wakley, "Middlesex Hospital," *The Lancet* (28 November 1868): 695.
[37] Wakley, "Paris," p. 575.
[38] James Grey Glover, "Carbolic Acid and Death after Amputation at the Hip-Joint," *The Lancet* (10 May 1879): 681–82.
[39] A. Pearce Gould, "Carbolic Acid and Death after Amputation at the Hip-Joint," *The Lancet* (17 May 1879): 718–19.

it."[40] He may not have realized just how far the diffusion of his own doctrine had gone. G. T. Wrench, who penned the first life of Lister a year after his death, was unequivocal when he wrote, "The year 1879 may be called the decisive one in the history of Listerism."[41]

The explanation for Wrench's assessment can be found in what another of Lister's biographers, Rickman J. Godlee, referred to as the "swan-song of the already dwindling race of pre-antiseptic surgeons." It was the address in surgery delivered by William Savory of St. Bartholomew's Hospital at the annual meeting of the British Medical Association, which was held in Cork that August. Godlee elaborated that before Savory had even given his speech "some curiosity was excited by the open secret that he meant to tackle the subject of antiseptic surgery." The suspicions were soon confirmed, but it also became obvious "that he had no real knowledge of what was going on in Lister's wards" and "that inflammation was common in his practice." As irrelevant as his presentation was, Savory's sentiments contained

> the views of a considerable proportion of the senior members of the staffs of the London and provincial hospitals at the time. Like a poultice, it warmed and comforted the soul of many a middle-aged man, who had begun to feel the discomforts of an undermined faith; though it almost made some of the younger men, to whom time passes but slowly, despair of the future.[42]

The Lancet was the only medical periodical which gave any credence to Savory's comments, and afterward, according to Wrench, it "delivered one more attack upon Lister before its compulsory capitulation."[43] That foray came in 1880 and lasted for the rest of Lister's career. It centered around the argument of whether an antiseptic or an aseptic approach was more practical, and Lister's leading antagonist was Lawson Tait. (See Figure 17.) Wakley ended 1879 by agreeing with Savory that "simpler plans" than the antiseptic method could render "enviable" results. In the three years prior, the number of deaths from "blood-poisoning" at St. Bartholomew's Hospital had been eighteen "after 1235 operations, and this is at the rate of 1.44 per cent." Those who adhered to "Listerianism" were asked to produce statistics as good and to explain how such success could be achieved "if the germ theory in its past or present state contained the truth, the whole truth, and nothing but the truth." Wakley perceived that Savory's lecture "came as a disagreeable surprise to the advocates of the antiseptic system of surgery."[44]

On the contrary, the shock came four months later in a meeting of the Metropolitan Counties Branch of the British Medical Association, which convened at St. Thomas's Hospital. Only one of the many surgeons present, Thomas Bryant, voiced his ability to "effect with the use of ordinary precautions . . . as good results as any of those who followed strictly Mr. Lister's method." All the others spoke favorably of the

---

[40] Joseph Lister, "A Demonstration in Antiseptic Surgery," *The Dublin Journal of Medical Science* 68 (August 1879): 97–98.

[41] Wrench, *Lord Lister,* p. 282.

[42] Rickman John Godlee, *Lord Lister,* 3d ed. (Oxford: The Clarendon Press, 1924), pp. 322–24.

[43] Wrench, *Lord Lister,* p. 283.

[44] James G. Wakley, "Antiseptic Surgery," *The Lancet* (16 August 1879): 246–47.

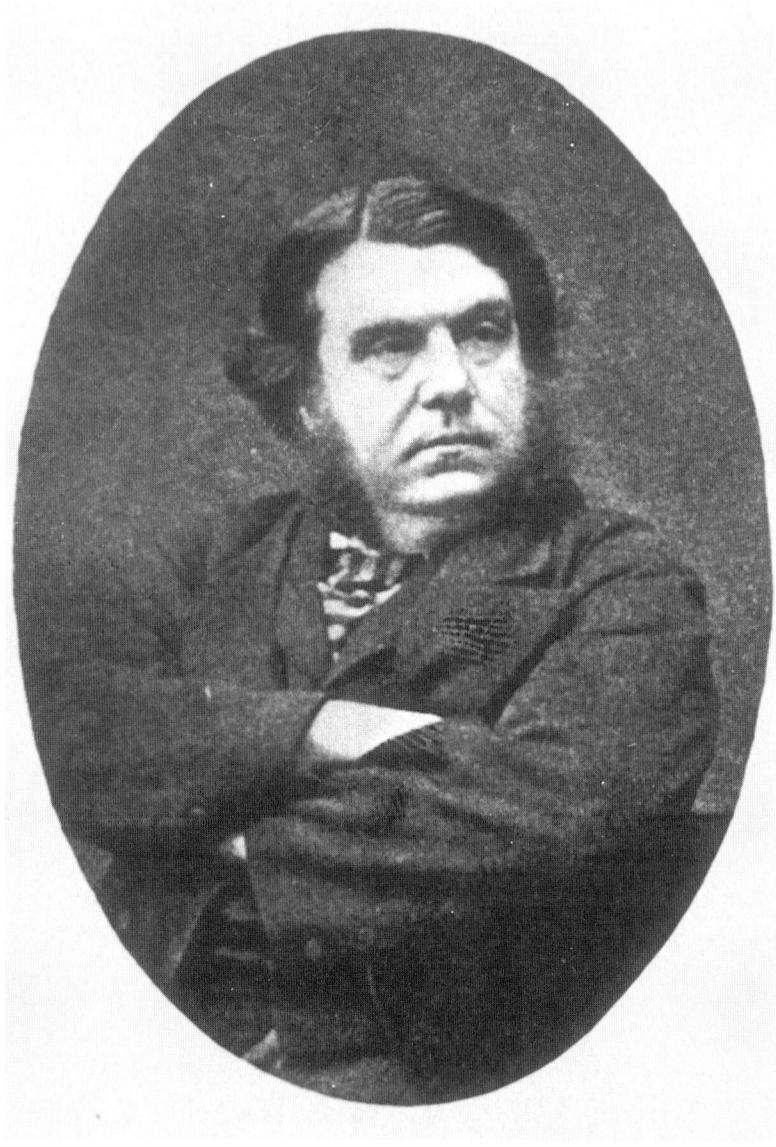

Figure 17. Lawson Tait

antiseptic principle, though Timothy Holmes did still reject the germ theory. Lister, who was in attendance, reacted to Savory and simply confessed that keeping statistics was not very high on his list of priorities. He also questioned the weight of Savory's figures, since they included the findings of other surgeons at St. Bartholomew's Hospital, like Thomas Smith who used Lister's technique "in many cases." Lister did enumerate the statistics pertaining to his surgeries, however, and stated, "I had six deaths from blood-poisoning in my 725 operations, or .82 per cent." He was offended that he had been accused of suppressing data and said that he could just as easily manipulate a lot of numbers as the few which he had supplied all along. To him it was a matter of trust either way, and he proposed that "one individual case, if it shows new pathological facts, is worth as much as a million."[45]

Ironically, on the same night that the discussion was held at St. Thomas's Hospital, the Midland Medical Society met to listen to a paper on Lister's method. The author, James West, was the senior surgeon at Queen's Hospital in Birmingham, where Lawson Tait practiced obstetrics. West began tentatively, observing that in "certain special surgical cases" the antiseptic technique was "preferable to all others." His true affection for Lister's system became clear, however, when he intimated that he favored it for "simple, incised, or lacerated" wounds. He then summed up exceptions to it by stating the ridiculously obvious. "We all of us know," he said, "that under the crudest, or, in fact, under no dressing, some wounds will heal." It went without saying that aberrations such as he described should never preclude a surgeon from trying antisepticism. West was also critical of Savory for proposing, in opposition to antiseptic practice, his own "plan of dressing," which was "merely a modified form of Listerism." He accused Savory of advocating "free ablution with clean water" while at the same time using one or more of Lister's materials, such as carbolized catgut ligatures or dressings soaked in partial solutions of carbolic acid. In response to Savory's desire for statistics, West rehashed the glowing reports from those in Germany who had used Lister's approach. To Savory's charge that other methods were cleaner that the antiseptic one, he answered,

> If Listerism has done nothing else it has secured an amount of attention that was never paid before to cleanliness; but it has done more, in that it has aimed at not mere prevention or removal of septic material, but at the destruction of it, by producing in the neighbourhood of all wounds an aseptic atmosphere.[46]

It was readily apparent that Lister's defenders were not going to allow others to receive his glory by promoting aseptic techniques, when it was the antiseptic system that had made such practices safe.

After hearing the lengthy breakdown of Lister's statistics, Wakley changed the rules of his game of numbers and qualified his position by adding,

> It does not seem to us by any means plain that the relative value of Lister's system as compared with other methods of dressing wounds can be determined by figures, but must rather be referred to the accumulating conviction of individual surgeons on the subject.[47]

Nevertheless, even Wakley could no longer resist the tide flowing in Lister's direction. A week later he wrote that the word "Listerian" would have to be used to distinguish

---

[45] James G. Wakley, "The Debate on Antiseptic Surgery," *The Lancet* (6 December 1879): 850–53.
[46] James F. West, "On the Surgical Cases in which Lister's Plan of Treating Wounds is Preferable to Any Other Method of Dressing," *Saint Thomas's Hospital Reports*, n.s., 10 (1879): 73–77.
[47] Wakley, "Antiseptic Surgery," (13 December 1879): 883.

the antiseptic practice from all other plans and that it was "destined to be the surgery of the future; for, however difficult the details or length of time required to carry out these principles . . . it must and will prevail, because it guards our patients from unquestionable dangers."[48]

Wakley attributed the swiftness of his change of mind to "a careful consideration" of a surgical illustration by Lister. The details of Lister's procedure were published in *The Lancet* on the same day that Wakley predicted the fate of antiseptic surgery. Lister had exhibited success in two particularly difficult cases, one of empyema and another involving a large open wound caused by the excision of a growth. The first of these witnessed the complete recovery of a patient whose pleural cavity had been incised by Lister more than three weeks before to withdraw "a large quantity of thick yellow pus." The amount of pus was so great that it not only vastly expanded the left pleura but also moved the heart "over to the right side, so that its apex beat at the right nipple." When Lister changed the dressing, it was dry, and all that remained in the silver drainage tube was some white lymph; he replaced India rubber tubes with metal ones after the first few days in such cases because of "the tendency of the thorax to contract on that side." The lymph obstructed drainage so that there was an ounce of "slightly tinged serous fluid" contained in the cavity, which had also been dry during previous dressings.[49]

The second of Lister's demonstrations which converted Wakley was the removal of a fibroid tumor from a patient's back. It was "firmly adherent to the spinous processes of four of the dorsal vertebrae." The hollow area left by the surgery was covered with skin from the right side, but too much movement by the patient broke some of the stitches at the bottom of the flap, creating "a circular opening about two inches in diameter." In spite of this there was no pus, even after twelve days.[50] Ostensibly, Wakley was finally convinced of the efficacy of Lister's technique because it made possible certain procedures that would have been unthinkable otherwise. Lister had explained his system in the largest city, to the most hostile listeners, and it was as if he was describing it for the first time. He did a very good job of outlining the steps of his method, but the same lesson had been taught many other times for those who had wanted to learn. Now, the least willing pupil, who had vacillated on both Lister's system and the theory behind it, graciously succumbed.

---

[48] Ibid., (20 December 1879): 914–15.
[49] Ibid., p. 914; Joseph Lister, "Clinical Lecture Illustrating Antiseptic Surgery," *The Lancet* (20 December 1879): 901–902.
[50] Lister, "Clinical Lecture Illustrating Antiseptic Surgery," pp. 903–904.

9. FINAL ASSIMILATION AS A FACTOR IN THE DIFFUSION OF LISTERISM

LISTER MAY HAVE EFFECTIVELY silenced his opponents after two years in England's capital, but there were still those who insisted that an aseptic technique was sufficient. By aseptic they meant simply cleaning their hands and instruments to keep from introducing germs to wounds. They also made it clear that their practice was not based on Pasteur's germ theory of disease. This was particularly true of many surgeons who performed operations on the abdominal cavity and was most clearly demonstrated in cases involving female reproductive maladies. Since that was the specialty of Lawson Tait, and since he had earlier taken up James Y. Simpson's mantle in opposition to the antiseptic system, the stage was set for one final contest in the assimilation of Lister's method.[1]

An Italian surgeon, who visited Lister's clinic at King's College Hospital in 1878, later commented on the attitude of his English counterparts toward antisepsis. Paolo De Vecchi of Turin sent a communique to an American colleague which related, "While in England I noticed a general indifference, if not opposition, to the Lister method, in some of the then prominent surgeons, especially were the gynecologists indifferent and in the case of Tait there was open opposition."[2] Regardless of how determined Tait was to divorce himself from Lister's practice, however, asepticism would not have been adopted extensively by the medical profession until the germ theory had been proved. By that time the antiseptic system had evolved to the point that the success of mere cleanliness in some surgeries could be explained, and in the years that followed it became a preferable method of wound treatment.

William Watson Cheyne, Lister's former student and assistant-surgeon, described Lister's method as "aseptic" after his mentor modified it further in the early 1880s. Cheyne succinctly defined the term as "any method of treatment which aims at and succeeds in *excluding* the causes of fermentations from wounds."[3] Lister had used the word himself in 1879, referring to an operation he had performed only one year after he first published his results with the antiseptic technique. Writing to Hector C. Cameron, he reminisced about surgery

> in the old days of carbolic oil, & the bones were divided with cutting pliers, an
> antiseptic atmosphere being provided by wrapping lint steeped in carbolic oil

[1] Luis H. Toledo-Pereyra and Marjean M. Toledo, "A Critical Study of Lister's Work on Antiseptic Surgery," *The American Journal of Surgery* 131 (June 1976): 741; for the analysis of a social scientist who agrees that the aseptic technique was not based on the germ theory but Galen's humoral theory, see Nicholas J. Fox, "Scientific Theory Choice and Social Structure: The Case of Joseph Lister's Antisepsis, Humoral Theory and Asepsis," *History of Science* 26 (December 1988): 368–71.

[2] Quoted in George David Stewart, "Lister the Surgeon," *Supplement to the Bulletin of the New York Academy of Medicine* 4 (January 1928): 164–65.

[3] W. Watson Cheyne, *Antiseptic Surgery: Its Principles, Practice, History and Results* (London: Smith, Elder, & Co., 1882), pp. 362–64.

round the blades of the pliers after they had been inserted beside the bone, the wound having been kept aseptic by free use of the oil while the incisions were made.[4]

In another letter to Cameron seven years later, Lister discussed how to steep his catgut ligature in "1 to 2000 corrosive sublimate solution a little before the operation commences, to make sure that it is perfectly aseptic."[5] Clearly, he recognized that wounds and the implements of surgery could be made aseptic, but he looked upon both as achievable only for brief periods during surgery.

A professor of surgery at Berlin's Charite Hospital, Ernst von Bergmann, supervised the implementation of the aseptic approach which evolved into the comprehensive one still practiced today. He had been a leading advocate of antisepsis, and asepsis was a logical result of Lister's principle for him. In 1886, his clinic began the use of steam for the sterilization of dressings, towels, and gowns, and the earliest trials with Robert Koch's tuberculin were supervised there in 1890. William Macewen of the Glasgow Royal Infirmary's dispensary pioneered aseptic garb by wearing a white apron that could be sterilized. A German surgeon in the city of Kiel, Gustav Neuber, boiled his gown and was the first to wear a cap in the operating room; he also "designed a dust-free ventilating system" for a private hospital he built in 1883. William Stewart Halsted of Baltimore's Johns Hopkins University Hospital asked the Goodyear Rubber Company to manufacture two pair of gloves for him in the winter of 1889–1890. He wanted them to be thin and to have gauntlets. The gloves protected the hands and arms of his nurse from mercuric chloride, the antiseptic in which she soaked surgical instruments.[6]

The most important modification that Lister made in the decade after 1879 was admitting that success could be experienced in certain operations without the spray, though he continued to recommend it as one more way to be sure that germs were kept out of wounds. Lister became willing to compromise on this point following Robert Koch's experiments with anthrax and tuberculosis, which decisively proved that specific germs caused specific diseases, that germs varied in potency, that some posed no threat at all to humans, and that they were not exclusively airborne. He now included changing water dressings frequently, cleaning meticulously, ventilating freely, and choosing candidates for surgery carefully as antiseptic precautions. Some have injudiciously interpreted this as a dishonest attempt on his part to include the achievements of those who did not employ his technique under his umbrella of antisepsis.[7]

The other changes Lister made after 1879 involved experimenting with new anti-

---

[4] Joseph Lister to Hector Clare Cameron, 22 March 1879, Joseph Lister Papers, Library, Royal College of Surgeons of Edinburgh, Edinburgh, GD5, 1.

[5] Joseph Lister to Hector Clare Cameron, 2 November 1886, Joseph Lister Papers, Library, Royal College of Surgeons of Edinburgh, Edinburgh, GD5, 137.

[6] W. J. Bishop, *The Early History of Surgery* (New York: Barnes & Noble, Inc., 1960), pp. 168–69, 173; Thomas D. Brock, *Robert Koch: A Life in Medicine and Bacteriology* (Madison, Wisconsin: Science Tech Publishers, 1988), pp. 199–200; Sherwin B. Nuland, *Doctors: The Biography of Medicine* (New York: Alfred A. Knopf, 1988), pp. 382, 414; Fox, "Scientific Theory Choice," pp. 384–87.

[7] Lindsay Granshaw, "'Upon this Principle I have based a Practice': The Development and Reception of Antisepsis in Britain, 1867–90," in *Medical Innovations in Historical Perspective*, ed. John V. Pickstone (New York: St. Martin's Press, 1992), pp. 40–43.

septics, which he had always continued doing, and adding a layer to the antiseptic gauze; the one next to the mackintosh was also colored pink so the dressing would not be put upside down. Eucalyptus and oxidized turpentine oils, as well as thymol, were all tried but apparently not for very long; benzoic acid had even been recommended by Charles Darwin in 1878. Not until 1883, though, when Koch distinguished germicidal from preventive antiseptics, did Lister begin to look for an agent that would substantially replace carbolic acid. He settled on a double cyanide of mercury and zinc because it did not irritate the skin and was not water soluble. "It was soluble in the mixture of serum and blood which came from the wound in sufficient amount to render it an unfit soil for the growth of bacteria."[8]

Yet, it was not Koch but Pasteur who provided the impetus for Lister's transition, in a paper he delivered to the French Academy of Medicine in 1878. It was entitled "The Germ Theory and Its Application to Medicine and Surgery," and its premise was so simple that many members of the British medical profession were hesitant to take the next step; they had just adapted themselves to Lister's technique, "If I had the honor of being a surgeon," Pasteur mused,

> imbued as I am with the knowledge of the danger of exposure to the germs spread on the surface of all objects, particularly in hospitals, not only would I use only thoroughly cleaned instruments, but, after having cleaned my hands with the greatest of care, I would subject them to rapid flaming, which is not any more painful than what a smoker feels when he passes a hot coal from one hand to the other. I would use only lint, bandages and sponges previously exposed to air temperatures of 130 to 150 C. I would use only water that had been heated to temperatures of 110 to 120 C. All that is very practical. In this fashion, I would only have to fear the germs in the air around the patient's bed. Observation teaches us every day that the number of these germs is almost insignificant in comparison to those that are scattered in the dust on the surface of objects or in the most limpid waters. It, moreover, would not interfere with the application of antiseptic bandages. In association with the precautions that I have indicated, these procedures could be simplified. Dilute carbolic acid could be advantageously substituted for the caustic carbolic acid, avoiding the disadvantage of its causticity to the hands and respiratory system of the operator.[9]

The evolution from antisepticism to asepticism in British medicine is subtle and a matter of degree. The chief defender of the antiseptic technique in England, against those who primarily used an aseptic approach in cases involving abdominal surgery, was J. Knowsley Thornton of the Samaritan Free Hospital for Women and Children in London. In August and September, 1879, an article of his entitled "The Antiseptic Method in Relation to Drainage of the Peritoneum in Abdominal Surgery" was published in three parts in *The Lancet*. It dealt almost exclusively with ovariotomies be-

---

[8] W. Watson Cheyne, *Lister and His Achievement* (London: Longmans, Green and Co., 1925), pp. 36–37; Richard B. Fisher, *Joseph Lister, 1827–1912* (New York: Stein and Day, 1977), pp. 260, 272–73.
[9] Karel B. Absolon, Mary J. Absolon, and Ralph Zientek, "From Antisepsis to Asepsis: Louis Pasteur's publication on 'The Germ Theory and Its Application to Medicine and Surgery,'" *Review of Surgery* 27 (July–August 1970): 246, 254.

cause they required drainage more often than other types of abdominal operations. The use of drainage tubes was one of the chief concerns of obstetricians because it provided easy access for septic elements from the outside, delayed healing, and often left a granulating sore where the tube had been. Also, the incision for drainage tubes herniated many times. Replacing glass tubes with those made from India rubber helped solve these problems to some extent because the rubber tubing could be shortened from time to time as the wound began to close from the inside.

Thornton, who had studied under Lister, recognized that many obstetricians and others who performed abdominal surgeries had initially feared that using carbolic acid on their hands and instruments would be more dangerous to the patient than germs themselves. They reasoned thus because the peritoneal cavity is aseptic under normal circumstances, and they were concerned about irritating it unnecessarily. By merely washing what came into contact with their patients, they could avoid that likelihood and keep the peritoneum free of germs as well. Antiseptic ovariotomies became accepted, however, because discharges from the peritoneum needed to be kept aseptic too until the patient had recovered. Also, an unhealthy or injured peritoneum lost its effectiveness in warding off infection and was aided in recovery by the use of antiseptics.[10]

Thornton looked upon the employment of Lister's system as a necessity for conscientious surgeons, not a convenience. He argued that since all the contents of the peritoneal cavity could not be known until it was entered surgically, the only safe thing to do was use antiseptics. Many women had ovarian cysts tapped, to remove excess fluid, before they ever required surgery. Tapping was not always done under the strictest antiseptic conditions. Therefore, the chances were great that surgeons would find putrefaction, and it would be too late to adjust to such a situation after an operation had begun. Thornton emphatically stated his belief that "we are now able to say we can perform ovariotomy with perfect antiseptic precautions, in any case in which there has been no previous tapping, or in which tapping has been performed antiseptically." His faith in Lister's technique was founded on personal experience with ninety ovariotomies, and he freely interjected that none of his "uncomplicated" cases had resulted in death during the time that he had used the antiseptic method.[11]

In his concluding remarks on the draining of abdominal wounds, Thornton maintained that "the need of drainage has passed away; at any rate, cases requiring it must be very exceptional." He only applied that dictum to "thoroughly aseptic" or "fresh" cases, and he insisted that antiseptics be utilized as in any other surgical procedure. He also mentioned Thomas Keith, calling him "a staunch advocate of drainage."[12] Keith was "the foremost ovariotomist in Scotland," to whom Lister "had sent his cases of ovarian cysts for many years." Keith had enjoyed phenomenal success in surgery before the birth of antisepsis but adopted Lister's practice soon afterward, in spite of Lister's objections. Following a brief trial with antiseptic precautions, he "discarded these quickly and returned to simple aseptic methods."[13]

---

[10] J. Knowsley Thornton, "The Antiseptic Method in Relation to Drainage of the Peritoneum in Abdominal Surgery," *The Lancet* (30 August 1879): 307–309.

[11] Ibid., (20 September 1879): 418–19.

[12] Ibid., (27 September 1879): 462.

[13] John A. Shepherd, *Lawson Tait: The Rebellious Surgeon (1845–1899)* (Lawrence, Kansas: Coronado Press, 1980), pp. 103, 105.

Lister later explained his original attempt to dissuade Keith from changing his method by pointing out that his machine for spraying carbolic acid "was as yet inadequate for the production of a cloud sufficiently large to cover the whole field of operation and sufficiently fine to avoid needless irritation." Lister believed that the amount of the acid absorbed had to equal or exceed the amount of drainage in order to prevent putrefaction from occurring. He also understood the reason Keith and others had such admirable results without the use of antiseptics. He wrote, "The answer is, I believe, to be found in certain peculiarities of the abdominal cavity." He specifically listed two of its characteristics, noting that when the surface of it is incised, plasma "is poured into a large cavity lined with a serous membrane disposed to absorb it as fast as it is effused. A further peculiarity in favour of abdominal wounds is due to the high vital power of the peritoneum."[14]

In the same month that Thornton's three-part article concluded, Lister was in Amsterdam for the International Congress of Medical Science. He had gone there to reply to those who still objected to antisepsis. He "was received," according to Ernest Hart, the editor of *The British Medical Journal,*

> by the whole Congress with an enthusiasm which knew no bounds. When he stepped forward to the desk to open his address (which was delivered, with but few notes, in improvised French), the whole assembly rose to their feet; and, with deafening and repeated rounds of cheers, waving of hats and handkerchiefs, hailed the distinguished Professor of King's College with acclamations renewed minute after minute, and time after time, as his name was again and again shouted forth by some grateful and enthusiastic acolyte. This remarkable scene— unprecedented, we imagine, in the history of medical science—continued for some minutes.[15]

The subject of whether or not antiseptics should be used was still being debated in England too, in cases of ovariotomy, and was taken up by the Royal Medical and Chirurgical Society in London on February 10, 1880. The purpose of the meeting was to hear a paper by Lawson Tait on the topic, in which he stated that despite his belief in the germ theory, he did not endorse Listerism in obstetrics. Tait alluded to pre-antiseptic success in ovariotomies and reported that Keith's mortality rate had decreased to between eight and nine percent. His own results with one-hundred such operations showed a nineteen percent death toll in the first fifty compared to three percent in the second. He assigned the exact same percentages to the findings of Spencer Wells, a gynecologist in London who had pioneered ovariotomy and had made it "an acceptable and reasonably safe procedure."[16]

Pertaining to Lister's guidelines, Tait concluded "that the recovery of his patients was not facilitated by them." He admitted being "strongly impressed" by the results of

---

[14] Quoted in Ibid., p. 104.

[15] Ernest Hart, "International Congress of Medical Science, Amsterdam," *The British Medical Journal* (20 September 1879): 453; Lister read and wrote French, in addition to speaking it extemporaneously, according to Fisher, *Joseph Lister,* pp. 203, 248, 293–94.

[16] Shepherd, *Lawson Tait,* pp. 154, 201–202; James G. Wakley, "Royal Medical & Chirurgical Society," *The Lancet* (14 February 1880): 250–51.

the antiseptic system at first and said that he would "continue to employ the antiseptic precautions during operation, unless a wider experience decided that they also might be given up." Without exception, those who replied to Tait had experienced "diametrically opposite conclusions." Among the respondents was Spencer Wells, who had already recorded better outcomes with antiseptics than without. He acknowledged that he "was considerably consoled" at the news that Tait was going to continue to operate under antiseptic precautions. He added that, due to the use of antiseptics, he had not "seen a single drop of pus" in his patients' wounds in two years. Wells also explained that he had to use ice to bring fevers down before the days of antisepticism but that fevers had not been a problem since. He ended his comments by citing the psychological benefits of Lister's technique, as well as the physical. "Under antiseptics," he stated, "the surgeon's mind is rendered easy; he has less occasion to visit his patient, he feels certain that recovery will take place with less danger to the patient, and he is freed from the anxiety which he used to feel."[17]

Tait clarified the extent to which he still used some of Lister's technique, and the only part of it he persisted in was "the spray, because he did not see that it did any harm, and it might possibly be of good." He followed up his remarks to the Royal Medical and Chirurgical Society with a letter to James Wakley two months later. In it he was extremely critical of antiseptic dressings, writing that they were "positively hurtful." He then elaborated, "In my experience it was an almost uniform result that wounds dressed after Lister's plan suppurated, and in many cases they sloughed; and though none of the patients died, many of the recoveries were anxious and protracted." To those who placed the blame for his failures on his "imperfect method of using the dressings," Tait retorted "that if the proper use of the dressings was above my intelligence, it was useless for general application."[18]

Eight months after Tait wrote to Wakley, there was another, much more divided, meeting of the Royal Medical and Chirurgical Society. This time Tait and Timothy Holmes spoke against the use of antiseptics in cases of ovariotomy, while Wells challenged their arguments. The debate was sparked by George Granville Bantock's revelation that the three highest temperatures Keith ever charted were from patients treated antiseptically. Bantock was a gynecologist at the same hospital where Thornton worked, and when he assigned all of the credit for the success of Listerian doctrine to ordinary cleanliness, the embers were fanned into a roaring flame. Seizing the opportunity, Tait conveyed that, "in a series of 137 abdominal sections, in which 48 were done with *extreme* Listerian precautions, and the remainder successively by the elimination, one after another, of these precautions," the temperatures of his patients went down correspondingly. Ultimately, "after reducing the strength of the carbolic spray to 1 in 150, he had finally conducted the whole of the process under a spray of water alone!"[19]

Wells took issue with Tait by reiterating his previous reasons for having used antiseptics the past two years and by stressing that "in forty-nine cases out of fifty so treated the wounds heal by first intention." Even though the number of his patients

[17] Wakley, "Royal Medical," pp. 250–52.
[18] Ibid., p. 252; Lawson Tait, "Lister's Antiseptic Dressings," *The Lancet* (24 April 1880): 666.
[19] Wakley, "Royal Medical," (18 December 1880): 976–77.

who died before and after he accepted Lister's principle remained at ten percent, he felt that these conclusions justified its application. Timothy Holmes, the London surgeon who had called for a comparison of the antiseptic technique to others when Lister moved to England's capital, did not agree. Since he still did not believe in the germ theory, he saw no difference in what was being espoused by the two sides. He admitted not understanding Lister's method, now that the details of it "had been so modified," and he questioned whether or not Lister did. He also objected to the notion that failures were due to a misunderstanding of the theory behind the practice, while successes were proof of it. "If this were all it came to," he reasoned, "and after the method had been so long in use there was still a quarrel as to its advantage in 1 per cent. of the cases, it might fairly be said that the theory was 'not proven.'"[20] (See Figure 18.)

Just as the discussion became more heated, Tait penned that the explanation for the different facts compiled would "be found in the peculiarities of the peritoneum." He confessed that his experience was limited to one field of surgery, but he repeated his contention "that as the quantity of carbolic acid used for the operation is diminished, so does the patient recover more easily, with less fever, distension, and sickness."[21] One of Tait's fellow-surgeons from Birmingham, Thomas Savage, reported his experiences with Listerian ovariotomy shortly after Tait's conciliatory admissions. Savage compromised also by stating that some of his fifty cases did take longer to heal than Tait's, but that due to using Lister's method he had only had two fatalities. He thought that the dressing delayed healing, not the spray.[22]

Savage was probably right, but antiseptic dressings kept micrococci from entering wounds, too. Interestingly, Alexander Ogston, a surgeon at the Aberdeen Royal Infirmary, submitted an article to *The British Medical Journal* two months later, in which he reported his success identifying certain micrococci as the cause of chronic abscesses, acute abscesses, and "blood poisoning." They appeared in all of the diseases, and he distinguished those that were organized in groups from those that were in chain-like arrangements.[23] For the former type he coined the term "staphylococci" from the Greek word for a grape cluster; the latter kind had previously been designated as "streptococci" by Theodor Billroth, the renowned abdominal surgeon from Vienna who pioneered the resection of the esophagus, segments of the intestines, and the pylorus. Billroth accomplished these noteworthy feats in 1872, 1878, and 1881, respectively, but did not adopt what he called "listering" until 1875. That makes his first achievement especially astounding.[24]

Ogston had been paid fifty pounds by the British Medical Association in 1879 to investigate the correlation between bacteria and hospital diseases. He had already constructed a laboratory on his own property to study the problem and spent the

---

[20] Ibid., p. 978.

[21] Lawson Tait, "'Listerian' Ovariotomy," *The Lancet* (1 January 1881): 35.

[22] Thomas Savage, "'Listerian' Ovariotomy," *The Lancet* (8 January 1881): 77–78.

[23] Alexander Ogston, "Report upon Micro-Organisms in Surgical Diseases," *The British Medical Journal* (12 March 1881): 369–70.

[24] Hubert Kunz, "The Reasons for Theodor Billroth's Initially Negative Attitude against Joseph Lister's Antiseptic Method," TMs, p. 2, Lister Papers, Royal College of Surgeons of England, London, Drawer 2, Envelope 2; Brock, *Robert Koch,* p. 80; Erwin Ackerknecht, *A Short History of Medicine,* rev. ed. (Baltimore: The Johns Hopkins University Press, 1982), p. 192.

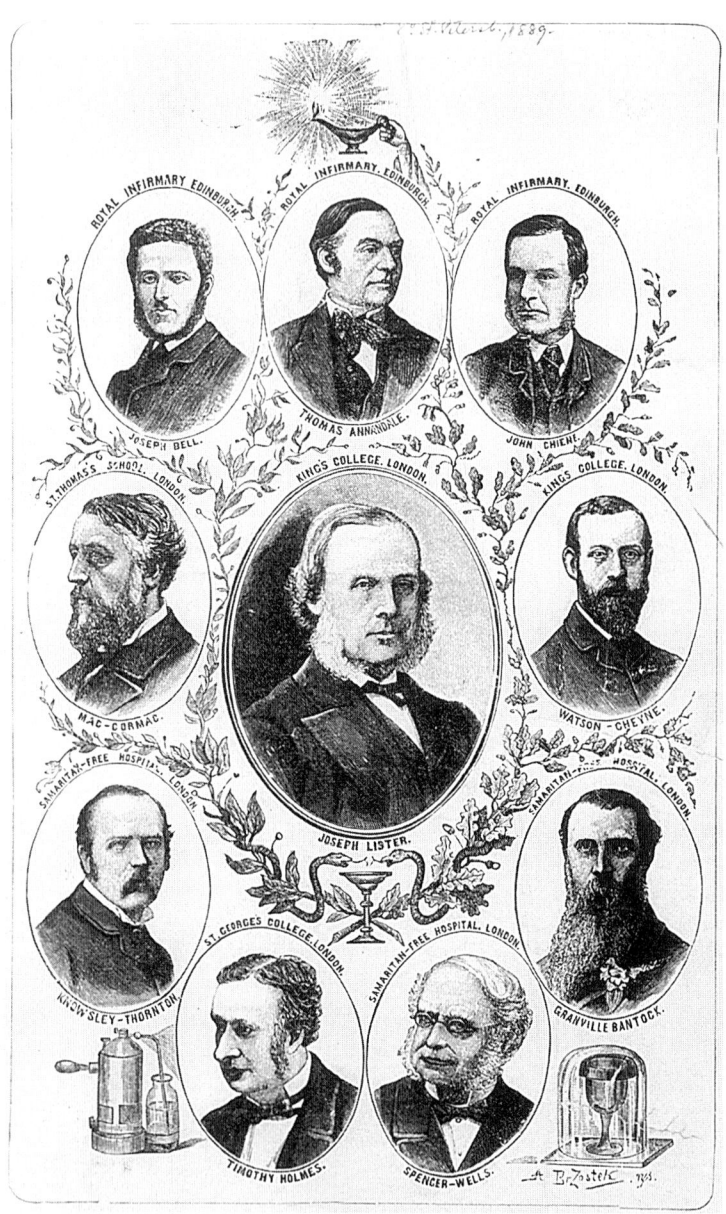

Figure 18. Lister and Colleagues

money he was given to buy a special microscope equipped with a condenser, a lens that could be used with oil instead of water for better magnification, and an incubator. Koch had relied on these instruments for his research, and Ogston followed his postulates carefully. By injecting guinea pigs, white mice, and wild mice with pus from abscesses that had infectious micrococci, he produced the disease in them. Repeating this procedure with freshly laid eggs, the shells of which had been cleaned with a carbolic acid solution before injection and were covered with antiseptic dressings afterward, rendered multitudes of the organisms but without any putrefaction; albumen taken from those same eggs, however, caused abscesses when it was introduced into animals. Ogston related his research to humans by studying normal and pathological body fluids, excised organs, and an amputated leg. He discovered that staphylococci and streptococci were never found in healthy specimens or diseased fluids in which there was no purulence but that they might multiply in a host's blood and cause death before an entry wound ever suppurated. Not only had Ogston conclusively established what the source of certain abscesses was, but he had also explained septicemia and how it could kill with no outwardly visible warning signs.[25] It should be remembered that Lister included abscesses in his first publication on the antiseptic treatment.

When Ogston's results were judged irrelevant by his colleagues and Ernest Hart, he decided to take his case to Germany in 1880, where he encountered an extremely receptive audience at the Ninth Surgical Congress in Berlin. Lister minimized the importance of his research, even though Ogston had visited him in Edinburgh and had introduced antisepsis in Aberdeen. This may have been because Ogston demonstrated that carbolic acid was ineffective when micrococci already existed in a wound. If it was applied before they gained access, however, it stopped them completely. Cheyne also took issue with Ogston, probably because the former had said that micrococci were innocuous, a statement which the latter reminded his readers of twice. Soon realizing his mistake, though, Cheyne credited Ogston with achieving the second greatest advance in the conquest of suppuration and septic diseases. Only antisepticism ranked as more important.[26]

Before the end of 1881, Lister voiced his opinion on the conflict over antisepticism that had been aired in the medical press for approximately two years. He had basically overlooked the combatants because "he rightly felt that he had said the last word and that Tait could be calmly and politely ignored."[27] Also, at the time the controversy was most intense, Lister received prestigious awards, which made opposition to his ideas all the more difficult. In 1880, he was awarded one of England's highest honors, the Royal Medal of the Royal Society, for his "numerous and valuable contributions to physiological and biological science during the last thirty years." The president of the society succinctly summed up Lister's accomplishment: "Condensed into a single sentence, the merit of Mr. Lister consists in the generalisation to living matter of the results obtained by . . . Pasteur with dead matter." That same year, Lister was also chosen president of the Clinical Society of London.[28]

When Lister did speak, it was to deliver an address on the treatment of wounds to the surgical section of the International Medical Congress; London hosted it in 1881. Exuding confidence in the wake of the recognitions that had been bestowed on

[25] Alan Lyell, "Alexander Ogston, micrococci, and Joseph Lister," *Journal of the American Academy of Dermatology* 20 (February 1989): 308–09; Ogston, "Micro-Organisms in Surgical Diseases," pp. 371–75; Brock, *Robert Koch,* pp. 65–69.

[26] Edward Kass, ed., "Classics in Infectious Diseases," *Reviews of Infectious Diseases* 6 (January-February 1984): 122; W. Watson Cheyne, *Suppuration and Septic Diseases* (Edinburgh: Young J. Pentland, 1889), pp. vi, ix–x; Ogston, "Micro-Organisms in Surgical Diseases," pp. 372–73.

[27] Shepherd, *Lawson Tait,* pp. 103, 105.

[28] Ernest Hart, "Professor Lister," *The British Medical Journal* (4 December 1880): 893; James G. Wakley, "Professor Lister's Recent Honours," *The Lancet* (18 December 1880): 984.

him, Lister rendered his own assessment of the efficacy of his system in obstetrics and gynecology. "The success which has attended antiseptic ovariotomy," he proclaimed, "has been regarded as a signal proof of the truth of the antiseptic principle." Lister emphasized that antiseptic surgery had made operations for small tumors possible before they became so enlarged. That would not have been thought of before the advent of Lister's method. He also judged that the lack of tension, after a tumor had been removed from a distended area of the body, nurtured healing, as opposed to the problem of too much tension in other wounds. He intended to continue using the spray, maintaining that as long as the machine was near him in the operating room, he would "not as yet dare to abandon it." Expanding on this sense of responsibility, Lister said that he "should not feel justified, except on perfectly established grounds, in omitting any part of the machinery by which results so important to our fellow-creatures have been arrived at." However, he did express the hope that he could one day forego its use, possibly by the next meeting of the congress.[29]

Lister became more animated as he talked, warning the medical profession that "we must not allow an exceptional case like ovariotomy to blind our eyes to the truth that the disasters of surgery in the past have been essentially caused by septic agencies." He extolled the virtues of the antiseptic system, reminding his hearers that "union by first intention has no longer the importance it used to possess." Furthermore, he proudly declared that in regard to "the essential points of avoidance of inflammation and fever, of pain and danger, it is a matter of absolute indifference whether primary union occurs or not." In a parting shot directed at the surgeons who had stopped using antiseptic dressings and had substituted an aseptic technique only, Lister asked what could "be more dirty . . . than a wound left covered up with the same dressing for weeks together?"[30]

The only practical distinction between antisepsis and asepsis was that one combatted germs chemically while the other did so thermally. The reason for the change was the implication that instilling "antiseptic agents into wounds was not enough and that total preventive measures must be invoked." Assuredly, surgical materials and instruments can be completely sterilized with heat, but the patient's skin and the wound itself are seldom free of germs. The belief that a perfectly aseptic operation can be performed is a myth. That the autoclave became available in 1883, however, made it possible for technology to establish the reality of the Listerian doctrine and permitted asepsis to surge ahead. Rubber gloves, surgical gowns, and protective masks soon followed as common attire in surgery.[31] Lister never personally endorsed these changes and was particularly vehement in his opposition to gloves. Only two years before his death in 1912, he chastised the once loyal Cheyne for making the transition to gloves. He lamented, "You must forgive me if I express my regret at what you say about the use of gloves; because it may convey to some minds the idea that you distrust carbolic lotion for the disinfection of the hands."[32]

---

[29] Joseph Lister, "An Address on the Treatment of Wounds," *The Lancet* (19 November 1881): 863–64.
[30] Ibid., (26 November 1881): 902.
[31] Owen H. Wangensteen and Sarah D. Wangensteen, "Some Pre-Listerian and Post-Listerian Antiseptic Wound Practices and the Emergence of Asepsis," *Surgery, Gynecology & Obstetrics* 137 (October 1973): 688–90.
[32] Joseph Lister to William Watson Cheyne, 5 January 1910, Joseph Lister Papers, Library, Royal College of Surgeons of Edinburgh, Edinburgh, GD5, 148.

The same year that Lister addressed the International Medical Congress in London, the Academy of Sciences in Paris presented him with six-thousand francs for applying the researches of Pasteur to medicine. Two years later, Lister was knighted as a baronet. The statements made by Ernest Hart, in regard to Queen Victoria's bestowal of such an honor on Lister, indicate that the full weight of his accomplishments was finally realized. Speaking of Lister, Hart summarized,

> His claims have indeed been universally acknowledged, and as enthusiastically by the profession throughout the European continent and America, as they are in this country. Listerism is a newly coined phrase, designating a principle and a method which are honourably known and gratefully remembered wherever men are engaged in any department of the profession in the effort to alleviate human suffering. It is not too much to say that the philosophical research and practical genius of Mr. Lister have revolutionised surgical practice throughout the world. On the battlefield, in the hospital, and in the homes of the sick, Listerism is a household word. The textbooks have had to be rewritten.[33]

In a magnanimous gesture, Alexander Ogston also offered his congratulations to Lister personally. With glowing respect and genuine affection, he wrote, "You have changed Surgery, especially Operative Surgery, from being a hazardous lottery into a safe and soundly-based science." He also called Lister "the leader of the modern generation of scientific surgeons." Ironically, as one observer has pointed out, it was Ogston who "finished scientifically" what "Lister started empirically."[34]

Lister continued to practice medicine for another decade, and he finally abandoned the spray in 1887. Ten years after giving up his trademark, he became the first member of the medical profession to be created a peer; he was ennobled as a baron on his seventieth birthday by Queen Victoria. William Gladstone "had proposed his knighthood tardily," but Lord Salisbury heartily recommended him for the peerage. Without any further controversy over the spray and with the passage of time, there was "no conflict between the aseptic and the antiseptic technique. The two were complementary and were often used together, depending on the circumstances."[35] As the famous physician, William Osler, once said, "It is the difference between tweedledum and tweedledee. They are both applications of the same principle."[36]

---

[33] Ernest Hart, "The New Baronets," *The British Medical Journal* (15 December 1883): 1207–1208.
[34] Alexander Ogston to Joseph Lister, 11 December 1883, Western Manuscripts, Wellcome Institute for the History of Medicine, London, MS 6970, 19; Lyell, "Alexander Ogston," p. 310.
[35] Jack Penn, "Lord Lister," *Medical Proceedings* 11 (3 July 1965): 300–301; Fisher, *Lister,* pp. 305, 311.
[36] Stephen Paget, *Pasteur and After Pasteur* (London: Adam and Charles Black, 1914), p. 40.

Conclusion

Joseph Lister was one of many people in the nineteenth century who experimented with new techniques. Had he been more aware of the obstacles others had faced in winning approval for their original contributions, he would not have been as shocked by the resistance he encountered. As has been noted, Lister had to be told about the germ theory and pleaded ignorance of the success in combating puerperal fever until after the triumph of his antiseptic principle. A book on the importance of carbolic acid as a disinfectant was in a second edition for three years before he learned of it, and drainage tubes had been introduced ten years prior to his employment of them. In addition, by the time Lister fathered antiseptic surgery the battle against anticontagionism had already been won, and hospital wards were better ventilated and less crowded than before. Specific diseases had even been linked to specific organisms.

That he admitted not knowing about at least four major breakthroughs in medicine and related sciences is a serious indictment of Lister. Due to the number of these apparent coincidences some have implied that he intentionally acted oblivious, presumably to secure his claim of independently arriving at the same conclusions and to assure his place in history. This second allegation is untenable because there is no evidence for it in the archives. After all, his own innovation far surpassed the others in terms of long-range consequences. The first charge is all the more disturbing, though, because three of the inventions were by Frenchmen, and Lister read, wrote, and spoke their language. He could have kept abreast of advances in their country. He was also in Vienna less than a decade after Semmelweis began washing his hands between patients, but must not have inquired about the reason for the drastic reduction in maternity ward mortality there. The most feasible explanation is that the attention he paid to his own researches and career kept him from noticing other matters of equal or greater importance before the advent of antisepsis.

Regardless of the reasons he was so uninformed, Lister was poised to apply the germ theory to surgery. More than a decade of practicing his craft as well as an intensive study of the analogies between inflammation and coagulation prepared him to make the connection between Pasteur's work on fermentation and infection in wounds. He also benefitted from sitting at the feet of surgeons like Liston and Syme, witnessing their successes with novel approaches to wound management. It goes without saying that if there had been no anesthesia, Lister's work would have been significantly hampered. Improvements in public health prior to the revelation of his system, and discoveries in bacteriology afterward, helped immensely also.

Lister was thus able to revolutionize medicine as a consequence of many factors. Make no mistake, though. He was the one who went through the birth pangs associated with the diffusion of a new idea, and his travail made operating rooms optimistic arenas of healing instead of pessimistic antechambers of death. It is also now clear that he began at least one aspect of his technique over two-and-a-half years earlier than has been recorded by his biographers. This is proof that he was refining his practice much sooner than previously believed and should give pause to revisionists who speculate that other developments such as better nutrition and strict cleanliness ultimately explained his achievements. Those who suggest that his thought was based on something other than what he said should be cautious, too. His legacy speaks for itself.

A re-examination of the controversy caused by Listerism seems especially poignant at a time when the world is struggling once again with nosocomial infections, increasingly resistant strains of bacteria, and incurable diseases of epidemic proportions. Possibly, a seed of intuition will be planted in the mind of a modern day Lister and that individual will be successful in dealing with the medical challenges facing humanity at the turn of the twenty-first century by learning how changes in tradition, theory, and technology were effected in the past. It is again "a time to heal."

Appendix A
A Chronology of Joseph Lister's Life and Career

1827	born on April 5 at Upton, in Essex, England, second son and fourth child of Joseph Jackson Lister, a Quaker and a wine merchant, and Isabella Harris Lister, a mistress of reading and writing at a Quaker school in Yorkshire who stopped teaching when she married
1827–1844	grows up in London where he studies the Latin classics and writes a number of papers on natural history; comes under the influence of Quaker ideas; learns to use the microscope with the help of his father, who had earned a fellowship in the Royal Society by improving the quality of lenses
1844	enters University College, London, because non-Anglicans are prohibited from enrolling in Oxford or Cambridge and completes a bachelor's degree in three years
1847	contracts smallpox, a year after his older brother dies of the disease, and suffers a nervous breakdown due to bereavement and the stress of his classes
1848	begins his training for the medical profession at the University of London
1852	graduates with a degree in medicine; becomes a member of the Royal College of Surgeons of England
1853	leaves London on the advice of William Sharpey, his physiology teacher, to tour other medical facilities; visits Scotland where he observes James Syme, the leading surgeon in the United Kingdom
1854	begins employment as a house-surgeon in Syme's wards at the Edinburgh Royal Infirmary
1855	becomes a fellow of the Royal College of Surgeons of Edinburgh and is appointed Lecturer on Surgery at the Edinburgh School of Medicine
1856	marries James Syme's daughter, Agnes, but not before resigning from the Society of Friends to join the Church of England; spends three months traveling on the continent of Europe with his new bride where he meets the leading physicians of the day; is promoted to assistant-surgeon at the Edinburgh Royal Infirmary
1858	publishes papers on the early stages of inflammation and the causes of coagulation, demonstrating that they are similar processes

1860–1869	moves to Glasgow to become Regius Professor of Surgery at the university there and is hired as chief-surgeon by the Glasgow Royal Infirmary
1864	is introduced to the writings of Louis Pasteur by Thomas Anderson, a professor of chemistry who also gives him his first sample of carbolic acid, a coal tar derivative, which was being used to treat sewage in Carlisle, England; accepts Pasteur's germ theory, which attributed fermentation in beer and wine to airborne microbes, and concludes that they also cause wounds to putrefy
1865	uses carbolic acid to prevent suppuration in compound fractures and is finally successful in healing the broken left leg of eleven-year-old James Greenlees
1867	reports the results of an additional year and a half of experimentation in *The Lancet,* England's foremost medical journal; defends himself against attacks by James Y. Simpson, the discoverer of chloroform, who attributes the first published reference to carbolic acid as an effective tool in combating putrefaction to Jules Lemaire, a pharmacist in Paris; denies ever claiming to be the first to allude to the said agent but does insist he is the first to use it to kill germs
1869	is grieved by the death of his father; reintroduces catgut ligatures but prepares them antiseptically; uses India rubber drainage tubes for the first time
1869–1877	is chosen to occupy the chair in systematic surgery formerly held by his father-in-law and is hired as chief-surgeon by the Edinburgh Royal Infirmary
1870	father-in-law, James Syme, dies; publishes a paper on the medical treatment of wounded soldiers in the Franco-Prussian War which comes too late to affect significantly the death toll but gains him wide acceptance in the German states and Denmark; mentions the carbolic acid spray in print for the first time
1871	operates on Queen Victoria to incise a large abscess in her left underarm
1875	accepts an invitation by the Congress of German Surgery to visit the universities of Berlin, Leipzig, and Munich, where he receives a conquering hero's welcome because of the phenomenal success physicians like Richard von Volkmann, who had no fatalities in his previous thirty-one cases of compound fractures, enjoyed with Lister's antiseptic technique
1876	journeys to the United States for its centennial and attends the International Medical Congress in Philadelphia, where he is elected President of the Surgical Section
1877–1893	assumes the chair of clinical surgery at King's College in London and begins his practice at King's College Hospital

1879	is greeted with a prolonged standing ovation at the International Congress of Medical Science in Amsterdam, where he replies to those who still object to the use of antiseptics in wound management
1880	is awarded the Royal Medal by the Royal Society
1881	is presented with six-thousand francs by the Academy of Sciences in Paris for applying the researches of Pasteur to medicine
1883	is made a baronet by Queen Victoria
1887	abandons the use of the carbolic acid spray
1891	plays a crucial role in helping to found the British Institute of Preventive Medicine which will be renamed in his honor twelve years later
1892	retires from teaching at King's College; attends Pasteur's seventieth birthday celebration at the Sorbonne, where the two men embrace
1893	ends his public career at King's College Hospital; loses his wife to pneumonia while vacationing with her in Rapallo, Italy
1895–1900	becomes the only member of the medical profession to ever serve as president of the Royal Society
1896	retires from private practice; is elected to preside at the annual meeting of the British Association for the Advancement of Science in Liverpool
1897	becomes the first member of the medical profession elevated to the peerage
1902	is consulted on the proper course to pursue in relieving King Edward VII's pain from appendicitis so that he can be coronated; is admitted to the Order of Merit as one of its first dozen members and is appointed to the Privy Council
1907	is presented with both the Freedom of the City of London and Glasgow but is too frail to make the trip north
1909	loses his ability to read and write; agrees to have his collected papers published
1912	dies on February 10 at Walmer, in Kent, England, and is buried beside his wife in West Hampstead Cemetery, consistent with his desire not to be interred in Westminster Abbey

Appendix B
A Review Essay on
Joseph Lister and Antisepsis

SINCE JOSEPH LISTER DID NOT WRITE any books himself, one must rely on his numerous published articles to find out what his views on antisepsis, the germ theory, and other issues were. They can be read in *The Lancet, The British Medical Journal,* the *Edinburgh Medical Journal, The Glasgow Medical Journal, The Dublin Journal of Medical Science,* the *Quarterly Journal of Microscopical Science,* and assorted other professional and specialized periodicals of the time. In order to honor Lister while he was still alive, *The British Medical Journal* [(13 December 1902): 1817–1861] did devote an exclusive number to the jubilee of his graduation from medical school. It chronicled his service to humanity and examined how the different branches of surgery had been affected by his technique.

Unfortunately, most of Lister's personal papers have not survived. A few are still in the hands of relatives in Great Britain, while others were given to the Library of the Royal College of Surgeons of England by Rickman John Godlee shortly after Lister's death. Included in the Library's holdings are three letters to Lister from Louis Pasteur and most of the ward journals from King's College Hospital. (See Figure 19.) The extant ward journals from Lister's years in Scotland are housed at the Glasgow Royal Infirmary and the Library of the Royal College of Surgeons of Edinburgh; the latter also has roughly one hundred and fifty of his letters, especially to Hector Clare Cameron and William Watson Cheyne. The largest collection of materials relating to Lister, however, is at the Wellcome Institute for the History of Medicine. Its Western Manuscripts division contains some seventy letters to Lister from his father, in addition to correspondence from his brother and other family members; Lister's medical school diploma, marriage certificate, and other memorabilia are there as well. The Institute's Contemporary Medical Archives Centre has two letters from Lister to Robert Koch.

A compilation of Lister's most important writings was supervised by Rickman John Godlee, William Watson Cheyne, Hector Clare Cameron, and others shortly before his death; Lister was physically incapable of directing the project himself because of poor eyesight, but he was involved in determining what should be included. The two-volume *The Collected Papers of Joseph, Baron Lister* (Oxford: The Clarendon Press, 1909) is the only contemporary source in book form. It contains a valuable introduction by Cameron and is a good place for researchers to find some of Lister's articles which are difficult to obtain.

A myriad of biographies on Joseph Lister exist, and with few exceptions they have been written by those in the medical field. Most of the studies are unduly laudatory because they were authored by those who were closest to Lister personally and professionally. Several biographies were published in 1927, the centennial of his birth, or in 1967 the centennial of his first article on antisepsis. Many articles have also been pub-

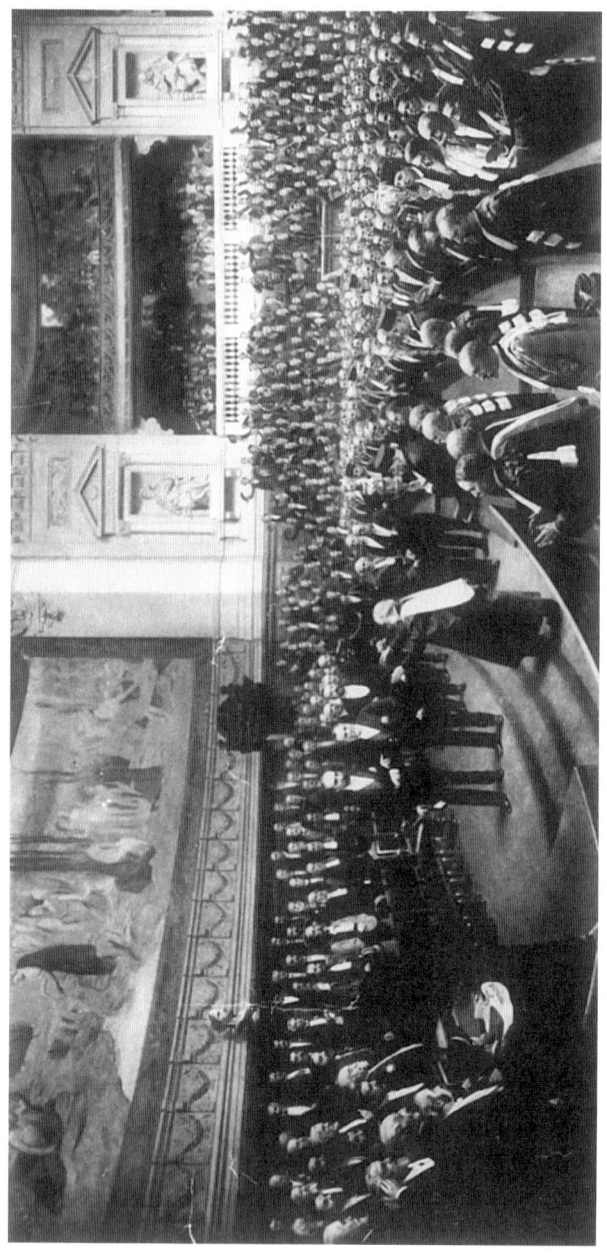

Figure 19. Lister embraces Pasteur

THE DIFFUSION OF LISTERISM IN VICTORIAN BRITAIN

lished on every conceivable aspect of Lister's life and work. It would not be feasible to deal with all of them in a review of sources, but collections of them for special issues as well as those that are particularly controversial will be examined. Most of those written from an historical perspective can be found in the following three journals: *Bulletin of the History of Medicine, Journal of the History of Medicine and Allied Sciences,* and *Medical History.*

Only three months after Lister's death, *The Canadian Journal of Medicine and Surgery* [31 (May 1912): 285–366] published a special issue devoted entirely to him, consisting of papers which had been read before the Academy of Medicine in Toronto on April 2, 1912. One of the selections had been written by Archibald E. Malloch, a house-surgeon for Lister at the time he began using carbolic acid as an antiseptic. The first book-length biography of Lister appeared one year after its subject's death. G. T. Wrench's *Lord Lister: His Life and Work* (London: T. Fisher Unwin, 1913) was penned by a physician in London who simply consulted the printed material on Lister. He concluded that Lister, not Hippocrates, should be recognized as the father of medicine because unlike the pagan he had God on his side; he also referred to Lister as a genius and a philosopher. Wrench's appraisal was definitely not very even-handed.

Four years after Wrench's book was published, however, the best biography for the next six decades was written by Lister's nephew and co-worker. Rickman John Godlee's *Lord Lister* (Oxford: The Clarendon Press, 1917) was based on his remembrances of his uncle as well as correspondence between Lister and other family members; also, letters from Lister to other prominent men in medicine and vice versa supplied Godlee with much of his material. Since Godlee was a surgeon himself, his work focuses primarily on the technical aspects of Lister's practice. He does credit Lister with causing a "modern revolution," and he spares no mercy in exposing those who made false accusations against his uncle or had a contrary spirit. Most subsequent lives of Lister have been based exclusively on Godlee. Cuthbert Dukes's *Lord Lister* (London: Leonard Parsons, 1924) is little more than an abridgement of Godlee for American readers, which he admits in his preface. Other titles that are essentially much shorter versions of Godlee include C. J. S. Thompson's *Lord Lister, the Discoverer of Antiseptic Surgery* (London: John Bale, Sons, & Danielsson, 1934), Douglas James Guthrie's *Lord Lister, His Life and Doctrine* (Edinburgh: E. and S. Livingstone, 1949), and Kenneth Walker's *Joseph Lister* (London: Hutchinson, 1956).

In addition to Godlee's book, which ran to a third edition in 1924, two other reminiscences by former associates of Lister were published in the 1920s. William Watson Cheyne's *Lister and His Achievement* (London: Longmans, Green and Co., 1925) is an honest appraisal of the contribution Lister made to medical science. It was the text of a speech delivered by Cheyne to the Royal College of Surgeons on the occasion of his acceptance of that organization's first Listerian Medal and Prize, and he included a eulogy to Godlee who had just died. Cheyne had served as president of the august body earlier and spoke on the need for more progress in medical care. He clearly intimated that Lister had not gone far enough. John Rudd Leeson's *Lister as I Knew Him* (London: Bailliere, Tindall and Cox, 1927) is undoubtedly the most biased of all the biographies of Lister. He compares his subject to Alexander the Great and Napoleon and finds them lacking. He also states that he felt "an almost sacred obligation" to acquaint his readers with the man he formerly served as dresser and clerk.

Coincidentally, he was obliged to fulfill his task on the one-hundredth anniversary of Lister's birth.

Other commemorative volumes also came out in 1927. A. Logan Turner edited *Joseph, Baron Lister: Centenary Volume, 1827–1927* (Edinburgh: Oliver and Boyd, 1927) for the British Medical Association; it contained several articles by men who had been house-surgeons for Lister. Furthermore, *Lister & the Lister Ward* (Glasgow: Jackson, Wylie and Co., 1927) highlighted the surgical wing in Glasgow where Lister plied his trade, contrasting operations before and after the introduction of his method and emphasizing the importance of proper hospital construction for maximum ventilation. A similar effort had already drawn attention to the method used by Lister for securing blood vessels. *Lister and the Ligature* (New Brunswick: Johnson & Johnson, 1925) was a monograph compiled by the research readers of the scientific department at the company which published the study; it stressed the correlation between the success of Lister's system and his improvements in the ligature of arteries.

A couple of special events that occurred in 1927 also merit acknowledgment. First of all, in October the American College of Surgeons, at its meeting in Detroit, displayed a collection of replicas of Lister's paraphernalia. It was furnished by the Wellcome Historical Medical Museum of London, where the originals were housed. After the meeting the items were permanently headquartered at the College's facilities in Chicago. The official festivities had been held in Lister's home city the previous April, but a bound catalogue was printed for the United States exhibition. *Lister Centenary Celebration* (London: The Wellcome Historical Medical Museum, 1927) contained a chapter by Hector Clare Cameron headed "A Short Account of the Evolution of Lister's System of Antiseptic Surgery." He was another student from Lister's days in Glasgow and also became a close friend, especially after Lister's wife died; Cameron had lost his wife too. Interestingly, his son, Hector Charles Cameron, wrote a biography of his father's teacher entitled *Joseph Lister: The Friend of Man* (London: William Heinemann, 1948). The second notable occurrence pertaining to Lister in 1927 was a symposium in his memory held at New York in November. Two months later a series of speeches from that gathering were published as a *Supplement to the Bulletin of the New York Academy of Medicine* [4 (January 1928): 133–182].

Two biographies of Lister for popular audiences were published prior to the centennial anniversary of his first article on antisepsis. Rhoda Truax's *Joseph Lister: Father of Modern Surgery* (Indianapolis: The Bobbs-Merrill Company, 1944) is the most readable of the biographies of Lister. Written by a woman known for her fiction, it is mostly a synthesis of the secondary literature on the man. There are no footnotes substantiating her assertions, but in that she makes Lister better known to the general public, her book serves a purpose. Laurence Farmer's *Master Surgeon* (New York: Harper & Brothers, 1962) is also very easy to understand because it is geared toward a juvenile audience. Again, there is no documentation, but Farmer does bring a doctor's point of view to his narrative, which Truax was not able to do.

Five years after Farmer's biography was published, the centennial anniversary of Lister's announcement to the world concerning the antiseptic principle was observed. The Wellcome Institute for the History of Medicine printed the proceedings of its Sixth British Congress which was held at the University of Sussex that September. F. N. L. Poynter edited the finished product which was entitled *Medicine and Science in the 1860s* (London: Wellcome Institute for the History of Medicine, 1968), and two of the papers dealt with antiseptic surgery and the role of Lister in the development of abdominal surgery, respectively. The former was written by F. F. Cartwright whose *Joseph Lister: The Man Who Made Surgery Safe* (London: Weidenfeld and Nicolson, 1963) incorporated the ward journals of King's College Hospital to shed light on Lister's practice. The latter was authored by John Shepherd who is better known for his biographies of Spencer Wells and Lawson Tait, two ovariotomists with very different views of Listerism. In April, 1967, the Royal College of Surgeons of England also sponsored a centenary conference to celebrate Lister's first published reports on the antiseptic technique. The result was an historical seminar, and the papers which were read were printed in a special number of *The British Journal of Surgery* [54 (Supplement 1967): 405–27]. One final memorial to Lister's debut article on the antiseptic treatment of wounds should be mentioned. *The Journal of Bone and Joint Surgery* [49B (February 1967): 1–23], in an addendum to its annual volume, featured two articles. One was an evaluation of the debt orthopedic surgery owed to Lister, and the other was a bibliographical biography of him. The latter, compiled by J. G. Bonnin and W. R. LeFanu, is particularly noteworthy.

Next, two efforts from the late 1970s need to be cited. Richard B. Fisher's *Joseph Lister, 1827–1912* (New York: Stein and Day, 1977) is the best biography since Godlee's. He writes with detachment, though sometimes in a cumbersome manner, and incorporates research from extant papers of Lister found in private collections. He also takes advantage of recently recovered parts of Lister's library which was sold by a public vendor in 1913. Fisher objectively concludes that Lister was one of a few people in the nineteenth century who led in the advancement of medicine founded on scientific principles. A. J. Youngson's *The Scientific Revolution in Victorian Medicine* (New York: Holmes & Meier Publishers, Inc., 1979) analyzes the intellectual origins of the introduction of anesthetics and antiseptics to medical practice. He relies too much on *The Lancet* to the exclusion of other medical journals, but his insight into the conflicts surrounding the reform of the medical profession is keen. The institution was jolted out of its stagnation by men like James Y. Simpson and Lister.

Finally, in the last twenty years several articles and chapters in edited works have been written which challenge the traditional interpretation of Joseph Lister and his contribution to the history of medicine that endured for seven decades after his death. The first volley fired in the attack on Lister was David Hamilton's "The Nineteenth-Century Surgical Revolution—Antisepsis or Better Nutrition?," *Bulletin of the History of Medicine* [56 (Spring 1982): 30–40]. The author, a member of the Department of Surgery at Glasgow's Western Infirmary, believes in a radical transformation of surgery during the 1800s but attributes sweeping changes to the improved general health of a well-nourished people. He contradicted himself, however, in the same year his article appeared. He co-wrote a chapter entitled "Surgeons and surgery" with Margaret Lamb for a book Olive Checkland and she jointly-edited, *Health Care As Social History: The Glasgow Case* (Aberdeen: Aberdeen University Press, 1982), in which he recognized the "pioneering work" done by Lister and that "patients under his care had a better survival rate."

Another inconsistent challenge to the innovativeness of Lister's method is Nicholas J. Fox, "Scientific Theory Choice and Social Structure: The Case of Joseph Lister's

Antisepsis, Humoral Theory and Asepsis," *History of Science* [26 (December 1988): 367–397]. He unequivocally states that antisepsis and asepsis were "parallel" developments and that to claim the latter succeeded the former is "myth." Nevertheless, he labels the Scottish surgeon, William Macewen, as the "first aseptic innovator," and Macewen was one of Lister's students in Glasgow who initially strictly adhered to the antiseptic technique before evolving an aseptic one.

The most engaging writings on Lister and his doctrine since his death are two chapters in edited works. In John V. Pickstone, ed., *Medical Innovations in Historical Perspective* (New York: St. Martin's Press, 1992) Lindsay Granshaw has written a chapter entitled "'Upon this Principle I have based a Practice': The Development and Reception of Antisepsis in Britain, 1867–90." Also, in Christopher Lawrence, ed., *Medical Theory, Surgical Practice* (London: Routledge, 1992) the editor and Richard Dixey have authored "Practising on Principle: Joseph Lister and the Germ Theories of Disease." Both selections argue the thesis that Lister's technique was one of several factors in eradicating hospital diseases and was probably less important than the following: simpler aseptic practices; new hospitals constructed after the pattern recommended by Florence Nightingale, with more space for each patient and improved ventilation; or better nutrition. Lawrence and Dixey also stress that Lister's disciples read back into his accomplishment an understanding of germs that the father of their thought could not have had when he began using antiseptics to prevent infection.

A chapter simply entitled "Joseph Lister 1827–1912," written by this author, addresses these attempts at revisionism and assesses Lister's historical significance. It is in volume seven of James A. Moncure, ed., *Research Guide to European Historical Biography,* 8 vols. (Washington: Beacham Publishing, Inc., 1992–93). Certainly there were other advances running concurrently with antisepsis, but to imply that they were more responsible than antiseptic surgery for the dramatic reduction in hospital mortality rates that occurred during the last third of the 1800s is presumptuous. Even the success enjoyed by some who used aseptic methods would not have had a scientific context apart from Lister's antiseptic practice and Pasteur's theory on which it was founded. To assume, due to the progress that has been made in the twentieth century, that asepticism would have inexorably led to an appreciation of bacteriology, in the wake of Robert Koch's isolation of the *tubercle bacillus,* is to do precisely what the followers of Lister have been accused of doing. The only way to assess properly Lister's place in the history of medicine is to interpret him, and whether or not he was original, within his own institutional and intellectual environment and in comparison or contrast to other practitioners of his day. He did not live and work in a vacuum, but like Isaac Newton, who applied the concept of gravity to the universe, Lister related the germ theory of fermentation to the cause of putrefaction in wounds. That was his singularly insightful deduction, and it has permanently changed health care.

Glossary *

abscess — a localized collection of pus in any part of the body, formed by tissue disintegration and surrounded by an inflamed area

acupressure — a method devised by James Y. Simpson for stopping veins and arteries from bleeding with strategically placed needles

albumin — any of several simple, water-soluble proteins that are coagulated by heat and are found in egg white, blood serum, milk, various animal tissues, and many plant juices and tissues

alimentary canal — the mucous-membrane-lined tube of the digestive system, extending from the mouth to the anus and including the pharynx, esophagus, stomach, and intestinal tract

anesthetic — any agent that causes unconsciousness or insensitivity to pain; they are usually given by injection or inhalation

aniline — an oily liquid derived from benzene, used in medical and industrial dyes

anthrax — an infectious, usually fatal disease of warm-blooded animals, especially of cattle and sheep, which is also transmissible to humans

anti-contagionism — a movement which opposed the belief that diseases were spread from one person to another; blaming bad odors and filth for diseases and advocating cleanliness for their prevention

antisepsis — the destruction of microorganisms that cause disease, fermentation, or putrefaction

apothecary — one who prepares and sells drugs and medicines; a pharmacist or druggist

asepsis — the state of being free of pathogenic organisms, infection, and any form of life

atomizer — an apparatus for converting a jet of liquid to a spray or vapor

attenuation — the process by which pathogenic microorganisms are made less virulent by being heated, dried, treated with chemicals, passed through another organism, or cultured under unfavorable conditions for them

bacillus — any of various rod-shaped, aerobic bacteria, often occurring in chainlike formations

bacteria — any of numerous unicellular microorganisms, occurring in a wide variety of forms, existing either as free-living organisms or as parasites, and having a wide range of biochemical, often pathogenic, properties

benzoic acid — a white, crystalline acid, with a slight odor, used in germicides and keratolytic ointments

bluebooks — official publications of the British government, so named for their blue covers

---

* All definitions, except those contained in the text of the book, come from Clayton L. Thomas, ed., *Taber's Cyclopedic Medical Dictionary,* 18th ed. (Philadelphia: F. A. Davis Company, 1997) and/or William Morris, ed., *The American Heritage Dictionary of the English Language* (Boston: The American Heritage Publishing Co., Inc., and Houghton Mifflin Company, 1970).

145

boric acid — a white or colorless crystalline compound used as an antiseptic or preservative

carbolic acid — a caustic, poisonous, white, crystalline compound derived from the distillation of coal tar or from benzene and used in various resins, disinfectants, and pharmaceuticals; also called phenol it is dangerous because of its rapid corrosive action on tissues

carbonate of lime — a salt of carbonic acid, the mixture of carbon dioxide and water, combined with calcium oxide

caries — gradual decay and disintegration of soft or bony tissue, or of a tooth, in pieces instead of large masses; as it progresses the surrounding tissue becomes inflamed and an abscess forms

catgut — a tough, thin cord or thread made from the dried intestines of certain animals, normally sheep, used for surgical ligatures

cesspool — a covered hole or pit for receiving sediment or drained sewage; also called "cesspit"

chirurgical — an archaic word, derived from Latin, for the practice of surgery; surgical

chloride of lime — a substance consisting chiefly of calcium chloride and calcium hypochlorite used principally as a disinfectant and bleaching agent

chloroform — a clear, colorless heavy liquid used in resins and as an anesthetic; first employed by James Y. Simpson to alleviate pain

cholera — an acute infectious epidemic disease, often fatal and characterized by watery diarrhea, vomiting, cramps, suppression of urine, and collapse

clinical surgery — operations performed on the basis of direct observation and personal medical attention

coal tar — a viscous black liquid obtained by the destructive distillation of coal, used as a raw material in drugs, organic chemicals, and ointments for skin diseases

collateral circulation — secondary or accompanying circulation, as in a side branch of a blood vessel

collodion — a highly flammable, colorless or yellowish syrupy solution of pyroxylin in ether and alcohol, used to hold surgical dressings and as a coating for certain skin diseases

comminution — the reduction or breaking of a solid body into varying sizes by grating, pulverizing, slicing, granulating, and other processes

communicable — able to be transmitted from one individual to another directly or indirectly

compound fracture — a fracture in which broken bone lacerates soft tissue and protrudes through the skin, or an external wound leads down to the fracture

compression — applying a soft pad of gauze or other material to the body to control hemorrhage or, moistened with water or medication, to reduce pain and infection

congeneric — resembling another in structure, function, or origin; two or more muscles with the same function

contagious — a disease that is easily transmitted from host to host by cutaneous contact or respiratory droplets

continued fevers — sustained fevers, as in scarlet fever, typhus, and pneumonia, with a slight daily variation in body temperature

contracted cicatrix — a reduced or shrunken scar left by a wound that has healed; it is less elastic than normal

cross-infection — the transfer of an infectious organism or disease from patient to patient in hospital wards, by those attending them or the air; nosocomial infection

curative — a remedy for an already existing medical condition; having healing or remedial properties

cyst — an abnormal membranous sac containing a gaseous, liquid, or semisolid substance, caused by developmental anomalies, obstruction of ducts, or parasitic infection

Darwinism — the theory that all organisms evolve from lower, pre-existing life forms and develop through the natural selection of variations that increase their ability to survive and reproduce

de novo — anew, afresh, over again from the beginning; to spring from a new combination of physical or chemical processes, not from living matter

diagnosis — scientifically and skillfully establishing the cause and nature of a pathological condition by evaluating the history of the disease process, signs and symptoms, and laboratory results

diffusion — the process of disseminating information as widely and as completely as possible

disinfectant — a term usually applied to a chemical or physical agent that kills vegetative forms of microorganisms; most are used on equipment and surfaces rather than in or on the body

dresser — one who prepares and applies dressings, protective or supportive, for diseased or injured parts

double cyanide — simply a combination of two cyanides; Lister used mercury cyanide and zinc cyanide as a non-irritating, insoluble antiseptic

embolus — an air bubble, detached clot, mass of bacteria, or other foreign body that occludes a blood vessel

empyema — pus in a body cavity, such as the pleural cavity or gall bladder

endemic — diseases that are peculiar to and recur in a particular locality

epidemic — diseases that spread rapidly and extensively among many individuals in an area

epithelium — membranous tissue, usually in a single layer, composed of closely arranged cells separated by very little intercellular substance and forming the covering of most internal surfaces and the outer surface of a body

epizootic — attacking or prevalent among a large number of individuals simultaneously

erysipelas — an acute disease of the skin and subcutaneous tissue caused by a streptococcus and marked by spreading inflammation

escharotic — producing or capable of producing a dry scab or slough on the skin as a result of a burn or by the action of a corrosive or caustic substance

ether — a volatile, highly flammable liquid derived from the distillation of ethyl alcohol with sulfuric acid, and widely used in industry and as an anesthetic etiology — that part of medicine that deals with the causation, origin, or reason for a disease or disorder as determined by diagnosis

excision — the surgical removal of an organ or part by cutting or as if by cutting

fermentation — any of a group of chemical reactions induced by living or nonliving ferments, such as yeast, bacteria, molds, or enzymes, that split complex organic compounds into relatively simple substances

fibrin — an elastic, insoluble protein derived from the interaction of fibrinogen with thrombin and forming a fibrous network in the coagulation of blood

first intention — healing that takes place when wound edges are held or sutured together without the formation of granulation tissue

fistula — an abnormal duct or passage from an abscess, cavity, or hollow organ to the body surface or to another hollow organ

fungi — any of numerous plants lacking chlorophyll, ranging in form from a single cell to a body mass of branched filaments that often produce specialized fruiting bodies, and including the yeasts and molds

fytte — a part or section of a poem or song; a strain of music; a canto

gangrene — death and decay of tissue in a part of the body, usually a limb, due to failure of blood supply, injury, or disease

genu valgum — a condition in which knees are very close to each other and the ankles are apart; knock-knee

genu varum — a condition in which the legs bend outward; bowleg; bandy leg

germ — a nonscientific term for minute organisms or agents, invisible to the unaided human eye, some of which are related to the production of disease

glycerin — a syrupy, colorless liquid derived from fats and oils, which is soluble in all proportions in water and alcohol

glycogen — a white, sweet powder mainly found in the liver, which is the primary animal storage carbohydrate; "animal starch"

granulation — the formation of small, fleshy, beadlike protuberances on the surface of a wound while it heals

guncotton — a pulpy or cottonlike polymer derived from cellulose treated with sulfuric and nitric acids, and used in the manufacture of collodion

hermetically — completely sealed, especially against the escape or entry of air

heterogenesis — the occurrence in certain organisms of alternating sexual (gametophyte) and asexual (sporophyte) reproductive cycles

histogenetic — the formation and development of bodily tissues, particularly the three primary cell layers of the embryo

histolytic — the breakdown and disintegration of organic tissue cells

holistic medicine — the comprehensive and total care of a patient, including physical, emotional, social, spiritual, and economic needs

homogenesis — reproduction by the same process in succeeding generations; the opposite of heterogenesis

hospitalism — a term coined by James Y. Simpson for the spread of diseases in hospitals through cross-infection

house surgeon — the senior surgical member of the hospital staff who acts in the absence of the attending surgeon

hygiene — the study of health and observance of health rules and the methods and means of preserving health

immunity — an inherited, acquired, or induced protection against a specific pathogen

incision — a surgical cut into soft tissue or the scar resulting from such a cut

India rubber — a light cream to dark amber, amorphous, elastic, solid polymer, generally prepared by coagulation and drying of the milky sap, or latex, of various tropical plants

infectious — capable of being transmitted through the invasion of pathogens without actual contact

inflammation — localized heat, redness, swelling, and pain as a result of irritation, injury, or infection

infusion — an admixture of soluble elements or active principles derived from steeping or soaking in cold or hot water without boiling

innovation — that which is newly created or introduced; a change in accepted thought or practice

inoculation — introducing the virus of a disease into subcutaneous tissue, a blood vessel, or an abraded or absorbing surface in order to immunize, cure, or conduct an experiment

invasive — tending to spread, especially as a malignant process or growth attacks healthy tissue, or a procedure in which the body cavity is entered

irritative fever — a disease characterized by or accompanied with irritation of the system or of some organ

lac plaster — a wound dressing made from the mixture of a pastelike substance and resinous secretions from the lac insect of southern Asia

laissez faire — the doctrine that government should not interfere with commerce

linseed oil — oil from the seed of the common flax which is used as a demulcent and emollient

laudable pus — the erroneous belief that a certain amount of pus in wounds was normal and healthy

ligature — a thread or wire for tying a blood vessel or other structure in order to constrict or fasten it

Listerism — the intricate system devised by Joseph Lister for preventing wound infection through the use of antiseptics, particularly carbolic acid

lying-in hospitals — health care institutions which specialized in treating prenatal and postnatal illnesses like puerperal fever

lymph — a usually clear, transparent, watery liquid that contains blood cells and acts to remove bacteria and certain proteins from the tissues, transport fat from the intestines, and supply lymphocytes to the blood

mackintosh — a patented, waterproof, rubberized cloth invented by a Scottish chemist

marine sponges — gauze pads made from the light, fibrous, connective structure of certain marine animals and used to absorb blood and other fluids, as in surgery and wound dressing

measles — an acute, highly contagious virus disease characterized by fever and the eruption of red spots over the entire body

medical wards — large hospital units where therapy with medicines is required, as opposed to surgery

melanuria — dark pigment in urine, one evidence of poisoning from too much carbolic acid

mercantilism — the theory of political economy based on establishing colonies for their raw materials and markets to attain a favorable balance of trade

mercury chloride — a poisonous, white crystalline compound, used as an antiseptic and disinfectant; also called "corrosive sublimate"

mesmerism — a theory of animal magnetism proposed by Anton Mesmer, which has come to mean therapy using hypnosis

miasma — a poisonous atmosphere formerly thought to rise from swamps and putrid matter and cause disease

micrococci — spherical, gram-positive bacteria whose cells occur singly or in irregular clusters

microorganism — an animal or a plant of microscopic size, especially a bacterium or a protozoan

midwifery — the practice of assisting a woman in childbirth, or the study of obstetrics

morphology — the science of structure and form of organisms without regard to function

mucilage — a thick, glutinous liquid obtained from certain plants containing gum, which is used as an adhesive

noninvasive — not tending to spread, as certain tumors, or a procedure that does not require entering the body, including puncturing the skin

nosocomial — pertaining to or occurring in a hospital or infirmary, as in cross-infection

occlusion method — completely sealing a wound with a covering to prevent infection from outside and to prevent inner moisture from escaping through the dressing

open method — allowing a wound to heal naturally by keeping it uncovered or exposed to the air

operating theater — a building or room for the presentation of surgical procedures to benefit medical students

osseous — composed of, containing, or resembling bone; concerning bones; bony

osteotomy — the surgical division or sectioning of bone; the operation for cutting through a bone

pandemic — a disease affecting the majority of the population of a large region or one that is epidemic at the same time in many different parts of the world

panspermatists — those who contended that spores, especially asexual ones, sprang from pre-existing life forms

paradigm — any example or model, particularly one that has been accepted as a standard by successive generations

patella — a flat, triangular bone situated at the front of the knee joint; "kneecap"

pathology — the scientific study of the nature of disease, its causes, processes, development, and consequences

peritoneum — the membrane lining the walls of the abdominal cavity and enclosing the viscera

physician — a person licensed to practice medicine; one who used to merely philosophize about disease causes

physiology — the biological science of essential and characteristic life processes, activities, and functions; all the vital processes of an organism

plague — a highly infectious, usually fatal, epidemic disease, especially the bubonic plague

plasma — the clear, yellowish fluid portion of blood, lymph, or intramuscular fluid in which cells are suspended; protoplasm or cytoplasm

pleural cavity — the potential space between the parietal pleura that lines the thoracic cavity and the visceral pleura that covers the lungs; it contain serous fluid that prevents friction

polymorphism — the occurrence of different forms, stages, or color types in individual organisms or in organisms of the same species

practitioner — one who practices an occupation, profession, or technique; a general term for all medical doctors

preventive — thwarting or warding off both mental and physical illness or disease; prophylactic

prognosis — a prediction of the probable course and end of a disease, and the estimate of chance for recovery

protoplasm — a complex, jellylike colloidal substance that constitutes the living matter of plant and animal cells, and performs the basic life functions

puerperal fever — septicemia or infection of the endometrium and of the bloodstream following childbirth; also called "childbed fever"

purulent — forming, containing, or discharging pus, the generally yellow liquid product of inflammation composed of albuminous substances, a thin fluid, and leukocytes; suppurative

putrefaction — the partial decomposition of organic matter by microorganisms, producing foul-smelling matter

pyemia — a form of septicemia due to the presence of pus-forming organisms in the blood, manifested by formation of multiple abscesses of a metastatic nature

pylorus — the lower portion of the stomach that opens into the duodenum, consisting of the pyloric antrum and pyloric canal

relapsing fever — any of several infectious diseases characterized by chills and fever, and caused by spirochetes transmitted by lice and ticks; also called "recurrent fever"

remitting fever — a fever alternately abating and returning, without intervals of afebrility, like malaria

resection — the surgical removal of part of an organ or structure, especially the partial excision of a bone

Royal infirmaries — small hospitals for the care of sick or infirm persons, funded by the British government

salicylic acid — a white crystalline acid used in making aspirin, as a preservative and flavoring agent, and in the external treatment of certain skin conditions

salubrity — wholesomeness; healthfulness; conducive or favorable to health or well-being

sanguineous — pertaining to or involving blood or bloodshed; blood-red

sanitation — the formulation and application of measures to protect public health; the disposal of sewage

scarlet fever — an acute contagious disease caused by a hemolytic streptococcus, occurring predominantly among children and characterized by a scarlet skin eruption and high fever

second intention — healing by indirect union or granulation which fills the gap between the edges of the wound with a thin layer of fibrinous exudate

septic — when an infection has spread from its initial site to the bloodstream, initiating a systemic response that adversely affects bloodflow to vital organs

septicemia — a systemic disease caused by pathogenic organisms or their toxins in the bloodstream; also called "blood poisoning"

serous — containing, secreting, or resembling serum, the clear yellowish fluid obtained after separating whole blood into its solid and liquid components

simple fracture — a break in a bone without rupture of ligaments and skin

sinus-forceps — pincers for positioning drainage tubes in wounds, made by grinding dressing scissors

sloughing — when dead tissue separates from the surrounding tissue of a living structure

smallpox — an acute, highly infectious disease caused by a virus and characterized by chills, fever, headache, backache, and widespread eruption of pimples which eventually blister, produce pus, and form pockmarks

spontaneous generation — the hypothetical development of living organisms from nonliving matter; abiogenesis

spores — an asexual, usually single-celled reproductive organ characteristic of non-flowering plants such as fungi; a microorganism in a dormant or resting state

staphylococcus — a term coined by Alexander Ogston for any of various Gram-positive, spherical parasitic bacteria occurring in grapelike clusters and causing boils, septicemia, and other infections

streptococcus — a term coined by Theodor Billroth for any of various round to ovoid, often pathogenic bacteria, occurring in pairs or chains

sulphate of iron — a salt or ester of sulfuric acid combined with iron for disinfecting and deodorizing

sulphite of soda — a salt or ester of sulfurous acid combined with sodium for disinfecting and cleansing

suppuration — the festering or maturation of a wound, resulting in the secretion of pus surgeon — a medical doctor specializing in surgery; one who used to practice the craft of surgery instead of merely philosophizing about illnesses and their cures

surgical wards — large hospital units where patients are prepared for surgery and subsequently have their surgical wounds treated

suspension — treatment using a hanging support to immobilize a body part in a desired position

synovial cavities — hollow spaces in the body containing the lubricating fluid of the joints

systematic surgery — operations performed on the basis of medical theories instead of empirical evidence and carried out with extreme caution

tallow — a mixture of the whitish, tasteless solid or hard fat obtained from animals and used in edibles or to make candles, leather dressing, soap, and lubricants

tapping — the puncture of a cavity with removal of fluid, as in pleural effusion or ascites; paracentesis

tar-bags — cloth containers of a dark, viscid mass of complex chemicals obtained by destructive distillation of coal, shale, or organic matter and used as antiseptics

taxonomy — the laws and principles of classification of living organisms into established categories

thorax — that part of the body between the neck and the diaphragm, partially encased by the ribs; the chest

thrombosis — the formation, presence, or development of a clot, which occludes a blood vessel or forms in a heart cavity because of coagulation

thymol — a white, crystalline, aromatic compound, derived from thyme oil and other oils and used as an antiseptic

transfusion — the direct injection of whole blood, plasma, or another solution into the bloodstream

traumatic fever — a disease resulting from wounds, especially those produced by sudden physical injury

tuberculin — a substance derived from cultures of the tubercle bacillus, used in the diagnosis and treatment of tuberculosis

tuberculosis — a communicable disease of man and animals caused by a microorganism and manifesting itself in lesions of the lung, bone, and other parts of the body

typhoid fever — an acute, highly infectious, bacterial disease, transmitted by contaminated food or water and characterized by red rashes, high fever, bronchitis, and intestinal bleeding; also called "enteric fever"

typhus — any of several forms of an infectious disease caused by microorganisms, carried by fleas, lice, and mites, and characterized by severe headache, sustained high fever, depression, delirium, and red rashes

union — growing together of severed or broken parts, as of bones or lips of a wound

vaccination — introduction of a suspension of attenuated or killed microorganisms into the body, incapable of inducing severe infection but capable of counteracting the unmodified species

vasomotor — pertaining to the nerves having muscular control of the blood vessel walls

ventilation — exposure to the circulation of fresh air for the purpose of retarding spoilage or the like

vestry — a committee of Anglican church members that administers the affairs of a parish or congregation

vibrios — any of various S-shaped or comma-shaped microorganisms which cause cholera

virus — any of various submicroscopic pathogens having the ability to replicate only inside a living cell

viscera — the internal organs of the body, especially those contained within the abdominal and thoracic cavities

vitiated — when the value or quality of something is impaired, made faulty or impure, or spoiled

vivisection — the act of cutting into or dissecting the body of a living animal, especially for scientific research

voluntary infirmaries — small hospitals for the care of sick or infirm persons, funded by private groups such as charitable and religious organizations

water dressing — a covering for wounds, introduced by Robert Liston, which is simply soaked in water

yellow fever — an acute infectious disease of subtropical and tropical areas, caused by a filterable virus transmitted by a mosquito and characterized by jaundice and dark-colored vomit resulting from hemorrhages

zinc chloride — a white granular powder, made by combining zinc and hydrochloric acid, for use as an antiseptic

zymotic — a term coined by William Farr for the analogy between fermentation and the chemical changes that occur in diseases; the process of wound infection

BIBLIOGRAPHY

PRIMARY SOURCES

ARTICLES

Annandale, Thomas. "Antiseptic Incisions an aid to Surgical Diagnosis." *Edinburgh Medical Journal* 20 (January 1875): 612–18.

Balfour, John. "Antiseptic for Country Practice." *Edinburgh Medical Journal* 22 (August 1876): 103–105.

Barton, John K. "Two Cases Illustrating the Advantages of the Antiseptic Treatment of Wounds." *The Dublin Journal of Medical Science* 61 (March 1876): 229–34.

Barwell, Richard. "Some Statistics of Antiseptic Operations in the Year 1877." *The Lancet* (2 March 1878): 306–307.

Bastian, H. Charlton. "The Discussion at the Pathological Society." *The Lancet* (20 March 1875): 409–10.

———. "An Address on the Germ Theory of Disease; being a Discussion of the Relation of Bacteria and Allied Organisms to Virulent Inflammations and Specific Contagious Fevers." *The Lancet* (10 April 1875): 501–509.

———. "Remarks on a New Attempt to Establish the Truth of the Germ Theory." *The Lancet* (5 February 1876): 206–208.

———. "The Bearing of Experimental Evidence upon the Germ-Theory of Disease." *The British Medical Journal* (12 January 1878): 49–52.

Bell, Joseph. "Cases Illustrative of the Antiseptic Use of Carbolic Acid." *Edinburgh Medical Journal* 14 (May 1869): 982–88.

Bennett, Edward H. "Report on Surgery." *The Dublin Journal of Medical Science* 48 (August 1869): 174–91.

———. "A Case of Empyema, Complicated by Pleural Fistula, Treated Successfully by the Antiseptic Method of Lister." *The Dublin Journal of Medical Science* 62 (November 1876): 361–70.

Bennett, John Hughes. "The Atmospheric Germ Theory." *Edinburgh Medical Journal* 13 (March 1868): 810–34.

Bickersteth, E. R. "Remarks on the Antiseptic Treatment of Wounds." *The Lancet* (29 May 1869): 743–44; (12 June 1869): 811–12.

———. "Carbolized Catgut Ligature." *The Lancet* (24 July 1869): 142–43.

Black, D. Campbell. "Mr. Nunneley and the Antiseptic Treatment (Carbolic Acid)." *The British Medical Journal* (4 September 1869): 281.

———. "Antiseptic Treatment." *The Lancet* (9 October 1869): 524–25.

Bryant, Thomas. "Professor Lister and Clinical Surgery in the London Hospitals." *The Lancet* (10 March 1877): 367–68.

Budd, William. "To the Editor of The Lancet." *The Lancet* (13 October 1849): 399.

———. "Investigation of Epidemic and Epizootic Diseases." *The British Medical Journal* (24 September 1864): 354–57.

Burdett, Henry C. "The Relative Mortality, after Amputations, of Large and Small Hospitals, and the Influence of the Antiseptic (Listerian) System upon such Mortality." *Journal of the Statistical Society* 45 (September 1882): 444–83.

Burdon-Sanderson, John. "The Origin of Bacteria." *The British Medical Journal* (1 February 1873): 120–21.

———. "Lectures on the Infective Processes of Disease." *The British Medical Journal* (26 January 1878): 119–20.

Callender, George W. "Two Years of Hospital Practice." *Saint Bartholomew's Hospital Reports,* 9 (1873): 1–46.

Cameron, Hector C. "Illustrations of Antiseptic Surgery." *The Lancet* (22 January 1876): 123–24; (29 January 1876): 165–68.

Chiene, John. "Edinburgh Royal Infirmary, 1869–1877." *The British Medical Journal* (13 December 1902): 1848–51.

Coats, Joseph, "Transactions of the Medico-Chirurgical Society." *The Glasgow Medical Journal,* n.s., 7 (January 1875): 115–21.

Craig, William, "Medico-Chirurgical Society of Edinburgh." *Edinburgh Medical Journal* 20 (July 1874): 69–75; (September 1874): 265–71.

———. "Periscope." *Edinburgh Medical Journal* 20 (November 1874): 461–69; 22 (November 1876): 461–68.

———. "Medical News." *Edinburgh Medical Journal* 21 (July 1875): 92; 22 (September 1876): 280–85.

———. "Correspondence." *Edinburgh Medical Journal* 21 (July 1875): 93–95.

Cresswell, Pearson R. "Case of Gunshot Wound of the Left Hip Treated on the Antiseptic Principle; Recovery." *The Lancet* (29 August 1868): 277.

Davies-Colley, N. "Two Cases of Varicose Veins of the Lower Extremity Treated by Excision." *Guy's Hospital Reports,* Third Series, 20 (1875): 431–35.

———. "Case of Partial Resection of the Head of the Humerus." *Guy's Hospital Reports,* Third Series, 20 (1875): 525–29.

Davy, Henry. "Five Cases Illustrative of Antiseptic Surgery and Pyaemia." *Guy's Hospital Reports,* Third Series, 23 (1878): 261–328.

Dewar, John. "On the Use of Carbolic Acid." *The Lancet* (14 December 1867): 757.

Ewens, John. "Use of Carbolic Acid." *The Lancet* (21 September 1867): 383.

Flaneur [pseud.]. "Antiseptic Surgery." *The Lancet* (5 January 1878): 36.

Forster, J. Cooper. "Clinical Records." *Guy's Hospital Reports,* Third Series, 18 (1873): 31–122.

Forward Progress [pseud.]. "Backward Progress: The Germ Theory." *The Lancet* (20 January 1872): 99.

Gamgee, Sampson. "The Treatment of Wounds on the Antiseptic Method." *The Lancet* (3 January 1874): 9–10; (10 January 1874): 50–52.

———. "Mr. Gamgee's Report on Antiseptic Surgery." *The Lancet* (24 January 1874): 143.

Glover, James Grey. "Carbolic Acid and Death after Amputation at the Hip-Joint." *The Lancet* (10 May 1879): 681–82.

Godlee, Rickman J. "On the Antiseptic System." *The Lancet* (17 May 1873): 694–95; (24 May 1873): 729–31.

Gould, A. Pearce. "Carbolic Acid and Death after Amputation at the Hip-Joint." *The Lancet* (17 May 1879): 718–19.

Harley, George. "Etiology and Clinical Bearings of the Germ Theory of Disease." *The Lancet* (4 June 1881): 903–907; (11 June 1881): 946–48.

Hart, D. Berry. "An Address on Pasteur and Lister." *The British Medical Journal* (13 December 1902): 1838–40.

Hart, Ernest. "Medical Society of London." *The British Medical Journal* (19 November 1870): 566–67.

———. "International Congress of Medical Science, Amsterdam." *The British Medical Journal* (20 September 1879): 453–66.

―――. "Professor Lister." *The British Medical Journal* (4 December 1880): 893.

―――. "The New Baronets." *The British Medical Journal* (15 December 1883): 1207–1208.

Haydon, William. "On the Antiseptic Plan of Treatment." *Edinburgh Medical Journal* 18 (March 1873): 792–97.

Hensman, Arthur. "On the Use of Carbolic Acid." *The Lancet* (14 December 1867): 757.

Hobson, L. J. "Antiseptic Surgery in Large Hospitals." *The Lancet* (8 June 1878): 851.

Hollis, W. A. "What is a Bacterium?" *The Lancet* (21 November 1874): 724–25.

Holmes, T. "Antiseptic Surgery." *The Lancet* (15 December 1877): 900–901.

Howse, H. G. "Two Cases of Internal Intestinal Obstruction Treated by Operation." *Guy's Hospital Reports,* Third Series, 19 (1874): 489–505.

―――. "On the Use of Carbolic Acid in Surgical Dressings." *Guy's Hospital Reports,* Third Series, 22 (1877): 506–507.

Hutchinson, Jonathan. "Carbolic Acid Treatment of Wounds." *The British Medical Journal* (4 September 1869): 269–70.

―――. "Dust and Disease." *The British Medical Journal* (29 January 1870): 118–19.

Keith, Thomas. "Antiseptic Treatment." *The British Medical Journal* (18 September 1869): 335–36.

Lamond, Henry. "Professor Lister and the Glasgow Infirmary." *The Lancet* (29 January 1870): 175.

Lawrie, Edward. "The Managers of the Royal Infirmary and Mr. Lawrie." *The Lancet* (3 July 1869): 29–30.

Lister, Joseph. "On a New Method of Treating Compound Fracture, Abscess, etc. with Observations on the Conditions of Suppuration." *The Lancet* (16 March 1867): 326–29; (27 July 1867): 95–96.

―――. "On the Antiseptic Principle in the Practice of Surgery." *The Lancet* (21 September 1867): 353–56.

―――. "On the Use of Carbolic Acid." *The Lancet* (5 October 1867): 444; (19 October 1867): 502; (9 November 1867): 595.

―――. "Illustrations of the Antiseptic System of Treatment in Surgery." *The Lancet* (30 November 1867): 668–69.

―――. "The Antiseptic Treatment of Compound Fracture." *The Lancet* (13 March 1869): 380.

―――. "Observations on Ligature of Arteries on the Antiseptic System." *The Lancet* (3 April 1869): 451–55.

―――. "Mr. Nunneley and the Antiseptic Treatment." *The British Medical Journal* (28 August 1869): 256–57.

―――. "On the Effects of the Antiseptic System of Treatment upon the Salubrity of a Surgical Hospital." *The Lancet* (1 January 1870): 4–6; (8 January 1870): 40–42.

―――. "The Glasgow Infirmary and the Antiseptic Treatment." *The Lancet* (5 February 1870): 210–11.

―――. "Further Evidence Regarding the Effects of the Antiseptic System of Treatment upon the Salubrity of a Surgical Hospital." *The Lancet* (27 August 1870): 287–89.

―――. "A Method of Antiseptic Treatment Applicable to Wounded Soldiers in the Present War." *The British Medical Journal* (3 September 1870): 243–44.

―――. "On Some Cases Illustrating the Results of Excision of the Wrist for Caries, the Treatment of Deformity from Contracted Cicatrix, and Antiseptic Dressing under Circumstances of Difficulty, Including Amputation at the Hip-Joint." *Edinburgh Medical Journal* 17 (August 1871): 144–50.

―――. "Professor Lister on Antiseptic Surgery." *The Lancet* (6 September 1873): 353–54.

―――. "Mr. Gamgee's Report on Antiseptic Surgery." *The Lancet* (17 January 1874): 109; (31 January 1874): 182.

————. "On Recent Improvements in the Details of Antiseptic Surgery." *The Lancet* (13 March 1875): 365–67; (20 March 1875): 401–402; (27 March 1875): 434–36; (3 April 1875): 468–70; (1 May 1875): 603–605.

————. "Demonstrations of Antiseptic Surgery." *Edinburgh Medical Journal* 21 (September 1875): 193–205; (December 1875): 481–87.

————. "Clinical Surgery in London and Edinburgh." *The Lancet* (31 March 1877): 475–77.

————. "Clinical Lecture on a Case of Excision of the Knee-Joint, and on Horsehair as a Drain for Wounds; with Remarks on the Teaching of Clinical Surgery." *The Lancet* (5 January 1878): 5–9.

————. "A Demonstration in Antiseptic Surgery." *The Dublin Journal of Medical Science* 68 (August 1879): 97–114.

————. "Clinical Lecture Illustrating Antiseptic Surgery." *The Lancet* (20 December 1879): 901–905.

————. "An Address on the Treatment of Wounds." *The Lancet* (19 November 1881): 863–66; (26 November 1881): 901–903.

————. "Remarks on Some Points in the History of Antiseptic Surgery." *The Lancet* (27 June 1908): 1815–16.

Littlejohn, S. G. "The Managers of the Royal Infirmary and Mr. Lawrie." *The Lancet* (3 July 1869): 29–30.

MacCormac, William. "On the Antiseptic Treatment of Wounds." *The Dublin Journal of Medical Science* 47 (February 1869): 52–62.

M'Donnell, Robert. "Observations on Traumatic Fever and the Treatment of Wounds by the Antiseptic Method." *The Dublin Journal of Medical Science* 48 (August 1869): 31–45.

Macewen, William. "Penetrating Wounds of Thorax and Abdomen Treated Antiseptically." *The Glasgow Medical Journal*, n.s., 7 (January 1875): 1–10.

————. "Lecture on Antiseptic Osteotomy for Genu Valgum, Genu Varum, and Other Osseous Deformities." *The Lancet* (28 December 1878): 911–14.

Maunder, C. F. "On the Antiseptic Ligature of Arteries." *The Lancet* (7 November 1868): 596.

Morton, James. "Carbolic Acid: Its Therapeutic Position, with Special Reference to its Use in Severe Surgical Cases." *The Lancet* (29 January 1870): 155–57; (5 February 1870): 188–89.

Nunneley, Thomas. "Address in Surgery." *The British Medical Journal* (7 August 1869): 143–56.

Ogston, Alexander. "Report upon Micro-organisms in Surgical Diseases." *The British Medical Journal* (12 March 1881): 369–75.

Paget, James. "Clinical Lecture on the Treatment of Fractures of the Leg." *The Lancet* (6 March 1869): 317–19.

Pirrie, William. "On the Use of Carbolic Acid in Burns." *The Lancet* (9 November 1867): 575.

Practitioner [pseud.]. "Mr. Lister's Antiseptic Treatment." *The Lancet* (30 October 1869): 629.

Ricketts, Frederick W. "On the Use of Carbolic Acid." *The Lancet* (16 November 1867): 614.

Roberts, Charles. "The Action and Use of Antiseptics in Surgical Practice." *The Lancet* (27 April 1872): 570–71.

Rose, John. "On the Use of Carbolic Acid in Compound Fractures, Wounds, Burns, and Gunshot Wounds." *The Lancet* (16 January 1869): 89.

Ryley, J. Rutherford. "Carbolic Acid in the Treatment of Compound Fractures and Abscesses." *The Lancet* (9 May 1868): 586–87.

Savage, Thomas. "'Listerian' Ovariotomy." *The Lancet* (8 January 1881): 77–78.

Seria mista jocis [pseud.]. "Antisepticism: a Fytte." *Edinburgh Medical Journal* 21 (October 1875): 376–382.

Simpson, James Y. "Notes on Acupressure." *The Lancet* (23 February 1867): 233–35.

———. "Carbolic Acid and Its Compounds in Surgery." *The Lancet* (2 November 1867): 546–49.

Smith, Thomas. "Clinical Lectures on Lister's Treatment of Wounds and Abscesses by the Antiseptic Method." *The Lancet* (25 March 1876): 453–55; (1 July 1876): 4–5.

———. "Professor Lister and Clinical Surgery in the London Hospitals." *The Lancet* (10 March 1877): 368.

———. "Conclusions from a Personal Experience of Lister's Antiseptic Treatment during Three Years of Hospital Practice." *Saint Bartholomew's Hospital Reports,* 14 (1878): 137–44.

Spence, James. "On the Use of Carbolized Catgut Ligatures." *The Lancet* (5 June 1869): 772–73.

———. "The Managers of the Royal Infirmary and Mr. Lawrie." *The Lancet* (26 June 1869): 888; (3 July 1869): 29–30.

———. "Carbolized Catgut Ligature." *The Lancet* (31 July 1869): 186.

Stevenson, Thomas. "Note on a Case of Melanuria." *Guy's Hospital Reports,* Third Series, 13 (1868): 407–10.

Syme, James. "The Managers of the Royal Infirmary and Mr. Lawrie." *The Lancet* (26 June 1869): 888.

Tait, Lawson. "Cases Treated Antiseptically on Lister's Method." *The Lancet* (14 January 1871): 45–46.

———. "Lister's Antiseptic Dressings." *The Lancet* (24 April 1880): 666.

———. "'Listerian' Ovariotomy." *The Lancet* (1 January 1881): 35.

The Times (London). 5 September 1882.

Thomson, George. "Antiseptic Surgery." *The Lancet* (20 September 1873): 432.

Thornton, J. Knowsley. "Antiseptic Surgery." *The Lancet* (27 September 1873): 470–71.

———. "The Antiseptic Method in Relation to Drainage of the Peritoneum in Abdominal Surgery." *The Lancet* (30 August 1879): 307–309; (20 September 1879): 418–20; (27 September 1879): 460–62.

"Translation of an Address on the Germ Theory [by Louis Pasteur]." *The Lancet* (13 August 1881): 271–72.

Tyndall, John. "The Germ Theory." *The Lancet* (12 February 1876): 262–63.

Wakley, James G. "The Surgical Use of Carbolic Acid." *The Lancet* (24 August 1867): 234–35.

———. "Carbolic Acid." *The Lancet* (28 September 1867): 412.

———. "King's College Hospital." *The Lancet* (12 October 1867): 455; (12 December 1868): 762–63.

———. "Compound Comminuted Fracture of Femur without a Trace of Suppuration." *The Lancet* (5 September 1868): 324.

———. "Antiseptic Surgery." *The Lancet* (17 October 1868): 520; (29 October 1870): 613; (16 October 1875): 565–66; (23 October 1875): 597–98; (16 August 1879): 246–47; (13 December 1879): 882–83; (20 December 1879): 914–15.

———. "St. George's Hospital." *The Lancet* (14 November 1868): 634.

———. "Middlesex Hospital." *The Lancet* (28 November 1868): 695.

———. "The Use of Carbolic Acid." *The Lancet* (5 December 1868): 728.

———. "Charing-Cross Hospital." *The Lancet* (9 January 1869): 47.

———. "University College Hospital." *The Lancet* (16 January 1869): 86–87.

———. "Report of the Thirty-Seventh Annual Meeting of the British Medical Association." *The Lancet* (7 August 1869): 211–16.

———. "Mr. Nunneley on Carbolic Acid." *The Lancet* (14 August 1869): 245.

———. "The Appointment of Mr. Lister." *The Lancet* (21 August 1869): 277.

———. "Mr. Syme on Medical Reform." *The Lancet* (15 January 1870): 89–90.

———. "Hospitalism and the Antiseptic System." *The Lancet* (15 January 1870): 91.

———. "Professor Tyndall as a Pathologist." *The Lancet* (16 April 1870): 555–56.

———. "Professor Tyndall." *The Lancet* (30 April 1870): 626.

———. "Germs." *The Lancet* (14 May 1870): 704–705; (19 November 1870): 714–15.

———. "The Antiseptic Principle in Surgery." *The Lancet* (17 September 1870): 411.

———. "A Sanitary Detachment on the Battle-Field." *The Lancet* (1 October 1870): 481.

———. "The Wounded About Sedan." *The Lancet* (8 October 1870): 517–18.

———. "Medical Society of London." *The Lancet* (29 October 1870): 604–607.

———. "Germs in George-Street." *The Lancet* (5 November 1870): 643–44.

———. "A Mirror of the Practice of Medicine and Surgery in the Hospitals of London." *The Lancet* (14 January 1871): 47–48.

———. "Provincial Hospital Reports." *The Lancet* (14 January 1871): 48–49.

———. "St. Mary's Hospital." *The Lancet* (1 April 1871): 446–47.

———. "Professor Lister and the Germ Theory." *The Lancet* (11 October 1873): 529–30; (25 October 1873): 600–602.

———. "The Debate on the Germ Theory of Disease." *The Lancet* (27 March 1875): 444–45; (10 April 1875): 514–15.

———. "High German Testimony to Antisepticism in Surgery." *The Lancet* (3 April 1875): 485–86.

———. "Pathological Society of London." *The Lancet* (10 April 1875): 511–513; (24 April 1875): 573–79; (15 May 1875): 682–85; (22 December 1877): 918–21; (17 May 1879): 703–705.

———. "The Germ Theory of Disease." *The Lancet* (15 May 1875): 694–95.

———. "Professor Lister in Germany." *The Lancet* (19 June 1875): 868.

———. "Clinical Society of London." *The Lancet* (16 October 1875): 561–62; (30 October 1875): 627–29; (20 November 1875): 737–39.

———. "The Debate on Antiseptic Surgery." *The Lancet* (20 November 1875): 743–44; (6 December 1879): 850–54.

———. "The Antiseptic Methods." *The Lancet* (19 August 1876): 267–68.

———. "Professor Lister." *The Lancet* (10 March 1877): 361.

———. "The Germ Theory and Spontaneous Generation." *The Lancet* (12 May 1877): 691–93; (16 June 1877): 886.

———. "King's College." *The Lancet* (6 October 1877): 488–89.

———. "Present State of the Bacteria Question." *The Lancet* (15 December 1877): 892–93.

———. "Paris." *The Lancet* (19 April 1879): 574–75.

———. "Organisms Under Antiseptic Dressings." *The Lancet* (17 May 1879): 710–11.

———. "Royal Medical & Chirurgical Society." *The Lancet* (14 February 1880): 250–52; (18 December 1880): 976–78.

———. "Professor Lister's Recent Honours." *The Lancet* (18 December 1880): 984.

———. "'Blood Diseases' and the 'Germ Theory'." *The Lancet* (2 April 1881): 546–47.

———. "The International Medical Congress." *The Lancet* (13 August 1881): 290–91.

———. "Bacterial Pathology." *The Lancet* (2 December 1882): 947–48.

West, James F. "On the Surgical Cases in which Lister's Plan of Treating Wounds is Preferable to Any Other Method of Dressing." *Saint Thomas's Hospital Reports,* n.s., 10 (1879): 73–83.

Will, J. C. Ogilvie. "Illustrations of Antiseptic Treatment in Minor Surgery." *The Lancet* (13 July 1878): 39–41; (20 July 1878): 78–79.

Wolfe, J. R. "On the Use of Carbolic Acid." *The Lancet* (28 September 1867): 410.

Wood, John. "The Address in Surgery." *The Lancet* (9 August 1873): 182–89.

Wylie, J. R. "Prof. Lister's Treatment of Wounds and Ulcers by Carbolic Acid." *The Lancet* (4 July 1868): 5–6.

BOOKS

Bastian, H. Charlton. *The Beginnings of Life: Being Some Account of the Nature, Modes of Origin and Transformations of Lower Organisms.* 2 vols. New York: D. Appleton and Co., 1872.

Beale, Lionel S. *Disease Germs; Their Nature and Origin.* 2d ed. London: J. & A. Churchill, 1872.

Budd, William. *On the Causes of Fevers (1839).* Edited by Dale C. Smith. Baltimore: The Johns Hopkins University Press, 1984.

———. *Typhoid Fever: Its Nature, Mode of Spreading, and Prevention.* London: Longmans, Green, and Co., 1873.

Chadwick, Edwin. *Report of the Sanitary Condition of the Labouring Population of Great Britain.* Edited by M. W. Flinn. Edinburgh: Edinburgh University Press, 1965.

Cheyne, W. Watson. *Antiseptic Surgery: Its Principles, Practice, History and Results.* London: Smith, Elder, & Co., 1882.

———. *Manual of the Antiseptic Treatment of Wounds for Students and Practitioners.* New York: J. H. Vail & Co., 1885.

———. *Suppuration and Septic Diseases.* Edinburgh: Young J. Pentland, 1889.

Duns, J. *Memoir of Sir James Y. Simpson, Bart..* Edinburgh: Edmonston and Douglas, 1873.

Gordon, H. Laing. *Sir James Young Simpson and Chloroform (1811–1870).* London: T. Fisher Unwin, 1897.

Lister, Joseph. *The Collected Papers.* 2 vols. Oxford: The Clarendon Press, 1909.

Lucas-Championniere, Just. *Antiseptic Surgery: The Principles, Modes of Application, and Results of the Lister Dressing.* Portland, Maine: Loring, Short, and Harmon, 1881.

Mumford, James G. *Surgical Memoirs and Other Essays.* New York: Moffat, Yard & Company, 1908.

Nightingale, Florence. *Notes on Hospitals.* 3d ed. London: Longman, Green, Longman, Roberts, and Green, 1863.

Paget, James. *Clinical Lectures and Essays.* Edited by Howard Marsh. New York: D. Appleton & Company, 1875.

Paget, Stephen. *Experiments on Animals.* With a Foreword by Lord Lister. New York: William Wood & Company, 1900.

———. ed. *Memoirs and Letters of Sir James Paget.* London: Longmans, Green and Co., 1901.

Pasteur, L. *Studies on Fermentation: The Diseases of Beer, Their Causes, and the Means of Preventing Them.* London: Macmillan & Co., 1879; reprint ed., New York: Kraus Reprint Co., 1969.

Paterson, Robert. *Memorials of the Life of James Syme.* Edinburgh: Edmonston and Douglas, 1874.

Richardson, Benjamin Ward. *Diseases of Modern Life.* New York: D. Appleton and Company, 1876.

Sansom, Arthur Ernest. *The Antiseptic System: A Treatise on Carbolic Acid and Its Compounds.* Philadelphia: J. B. Lippincott and Co., 1871.

Simon, John. *English Sanitary Institutions.* London: Cassell & Company, Limited, 1890.

Snow, John. *On the Mode of Communication of Cholera.* 2d ed. London: John Churchill, 1855; reprint ed., New York: The Commonwealth Fund, 1936.

Tyndall, John. *Fragments of Science.* 2 vols. New York: D. Appleton and Company, 1898.

LETTERS

Lister, Joseph Jackson to Joseph Lister, 4 December 1867. Western Manuscripts, Wellcome Institute for the History of Medicine, London, MS 6965, 55.

Lister, Joseph Jackson to Joseph Lister, 20 March 1868. Western Manuscripts, Wellcome Institute for the History of Medicine, London, MS 6965, 59.

Lister, Joseph Jackson to Joseph Lister, 10 November 1868. Western Manuscripts, Wellcome Institute for the History of Medicine, London, MS 6965, 61.

Lister, Joseph Jackson to Joseph Lister, 27 January 1869. Western Manuscripts, Wellcome Institute for the History of Medicine, London, MS 6965, 63.

Lister, Joseph Jackson to Joseph Lister, 6 June 1869. Western Manuscripts, Wellcome Institute for the History of Medicine, London, MS 6965, 67.

Pasteur, Louis to Joseph Lister, 27 February 1874. (photocopy). Western Manuscripts, Wellcome Institute for the History of Medicine, London, MS 6970, 11.

Lister, Joseph to Arthur Lister, 27 February 1877. Western Manuscripts, Wellcome Institute for the History of Medicine, London, MS 6968, 6.

Lister, Joseph to Robert Davidson Murray, 8 March 1877. Lister Papers, Library, Royal College of Surgeons of England, London, Drawer 5.

Lister, Joseph to Ernest Hart, 28 March 1877. Western Manuscripts, Wellcome Institute for the History of Medicine, London, MS 5424, 8.

Lister, Joseph to Hector Clare Cameron, 22 March 1879. Joseph Lister Papers, Library, Royal College of Surgeons of Edinburgh, Edinburgh, GD5, 1.

Ogston, Alexander to Joseph Lister, 11 December 1883. Western Manuscripts, Wellcome Institute for the History of Medicine, London, MS 6970, 19.

Lister, Joseph to Hector Clare Cameron, 2 November 1886. Joseph Lister Papers, Library, Royal College of Surgeons of Edinburgh, Edinburgh, GD5, 137.

Lister, Joseph to Hector Clare Cameron, 21 January 1907. Joseph Lister Papers, Library, Royal College of Surgeons of Edinburgh, Edinburgh, GD5, 65.

Lister, Joseph to Hector Clare Cameron, 19 February 1907. Joseph Lister Papers, Library, Royal College of Surgeons of Edinburgh, Edinburgh, GD5, 67.

Lister, Joseph to Hector Clare Cameron, 20 January 1908. Joseph Lister Papers, Library, Royal College of Surgeons of Edinburgh, Edinburgh, GD5, 90.

Lister, Joseph to William Watson Cheyne, 5 January 1910. Joseph Lister Papers, Library, Royal College of Surgeons of Edinburgh, Edinburgh, GD5, 148.

Secondary Sources

ARTICLES

Absolon, Karel B.; Absolon, Mary J.; and Zientek, Ralph. "From Antisepsis to Asepsis: Louis Pasteur's publication on 'The Germ Theory and Its Application to Medicine and Surgery.'" *Review of Surgery* 27 (July–August 1970): 245–258.

Ackerknecht, Erwin H. "Anticontagionism between 1821 and 1867." *Bulletin of the History of Medicine* 22 (September–October 1948): 562–93.

Ben-David, Joseph. "Roles and Innovations in Medicine." *The American Journal of Sociology* 65 (May 1960): 557–68.

Bonnin, J. G., and LeFanu, W. R. "Joseph Lister, 1827–1912: A Bibliographical Biography." *The Journal of Bone and Joint Surgery* 49B (February 1967): 4–23.

Brand, Jeanne L. "John Simon and the Local Government Board Bureaucrats, 1871–1876." *Bulletin of the History of Medicine* 37 (March–April 1963): 184–94.

Cartwright, F. F. "Lister—The Man." *The British Journal of Surgery* 54 (Supplement 1967): 405–10.

Churchill, Edward D. "The Pandemic of Wound Infection in Hospitals: Studies in the History of Wound Healing." *Journal of the History of Medicine and Allied Sciences* 20 (October 1965): 390–404.

Cowen, David L. "Liberty, Laissez-Faire and Licensure in Nineteenth Century Britain." *Bulletin of the History of Medicine* 43 (January-February 1969): 30–40.

Crellin, J. K. "The Problem of Heat Resistance of Micro-Organisms in the British Spontaneous Generation Controversies of 1860–1880." *Medical History* 10 (January 1966): 50–59.

Edgar, Irving I. "Modern Surgery and Lord Lister." *Journal of the History of Medicine and Allied Sciences* 16 (April 1961): 145–60.

Eyler, John M. "Mortality Statistics and Victorian Health Policy: Program and Criticism." *Bulletin of the History of Medicine* 50 (Fall 1976): 335–55.

Fox, Nicholas J. "Scientific Theory Choice and Social Structure: The Case of Joseph Lister's Antisepsis, Humoral Theory and Asepsis." *History of Science* 26 (December 1988): 367–97.

Geison, Gerald L. "Social and Institutional Factors in the Stagnancy of English Physiology, 1840–1870." *Bulletin of the History of Medicine* 46 (January–February 1972): 30–58.

Gibson, T. "Evolution of catgut ligatures: the endeavours and success of Joseph Lister and William Macewen." *The British Journal of Surgery* 77 (July 1990): 824–25.

Goldenberg, Ira S. "Joseph Lister: Innovation and Insurgency in Surgery." *Connecticut Medicine* 40 (November 1976): 771–73.

Hamilton, David. "The Nineteenth-Century Surgical Revolution—Antisepsis or Better Nutrition?" *Bulletin of the History of Medicine* 56 (Spring 1982): 30–40.

Hamlin, Christopher. "Providence and Putrefaction: Victorian Sanitarians and the Natural Theology of Health and Disease." *Victorian Studies* 28 (Spring 1985): 381–411.

Howie, W. B., and Black, S. A. B. "Sidelights on Lister: A Patient's Account of Lister's Care." *Journal of the History of Medicine and Allied Sciences* 32 (July 1977): 239–51.

Kass, Edward, ed. "Classics in Infectious Diseases." *Reviews of Infectious Diseases* 6 (January–February 1984): 122–28.

King, Lester S. "Germ Theory and Its Influence." *The Journal of the American Medical Association* 249 (11 February 1983): 794–98.

Larson, Elaine. "Innovations in Health Care: Antisepsis as a Case Study." *American Journal of Public Health* 79 (January 1989): 92–99.

Lidwell, O. M. "Joseph Lister and Infection from the Air." *Epidemiology and Infection* 99 (1987): 569–78.

Lilienfeld, David E. "'The Greening of Epidemiology': Sanitary Physicians and the London Epidemiological Society (1830–1870)." *Bulletin of the History of Medicine* 52 (Winter 1978): 503–28.

Linder, Fritz, and Forrest, Hugh. "The Propagation of Lister's Ideas." *Surgery, Gynecology & Obstetrics* 132 (November 1968): 1081–86.

Lyell, Alan. "Alexander Ogston, micrococci, and Joseph Lister." *Journal of the American Academy of Dermatology* 20 (February 1989): 302–10.

Malloch, Archibald E. "Some Memories of Mr. Lister." *Canadian Journal of Medicine and Surgery* 31 (May 1912): 48–53.

Malloch, Archibald. "Biographical Sketch and Memorabilia of Lister." *Supplement to the Bulletin of the New York Academy of Medicine* 4 (January 1928): 133–147.

Mason, Michael L. "Joseph Lister: Hospitalism and the Antiseptic Principle." *Quarterly Bulletin of Northwestern University Medical School* 33 (Spring 1959): 152–69.

Novak, Steven J. "Professionalism and Bureaucracy: English Doctors and the Victorian Public Health Administration." *Journal of Social History* 6 (Summer 1973): 440–62.

Ozer, Mark N. "The British Vivisection Controversy." *Bulletin of the History of Medicine* 40 (March–April 1966): 158–67.

Parsons, Gail Pat. "The British Medical Profession and Contagion Theory: Puerperal Fever as a Case Study, 1830–1860." *Medical History* 22 (April 1978): 138–50.

Penn, Jack. "Lord Lister." *Medical Proceedings* 11 (3 July 1965): 291–302.

Pennington, Carolyn I. "Mortality and Medical Care in Nineteenth-Century Glasgow." *Medical History* 23 (October 1979): 442–50.

Selwyn, S. "Sir James Simpson and Hospital Cross-Infection." *Medical History* 9 (July 1965): 241–48.

Stevenson, Lloyd G. "Science down the Drain: On the Hostility of Certain Sanitarians to Animal Experimentation, Bacteriology and Immunology." *Bulletin of the History of Medicine* 29 (January–February 1955): 1–26.

Stewart, George David. "Lister the Surgeon." *Supplement to the Bulletin of the New York Academy of Medicine* 4 (January 1928): 159–167.

Toledo-Pereyra, Luis H., and Toledo, Marjean M. "A Critical Study of Lister's Work on Antiseptic Surgery." *The American Journal of Surgery* 131 (June 1976): 736–44.

Upmalis, I. H. "The Introduction of Lister's Treatment in Germany." *Bulletin of the History of Medicine* 42 (May–June 1968): 221–40.

Wangensteen, Owen H.; Smith, Jacqueline; and Wangensteen, Sarah D. "Some Highlights in the History of Amputation Reflecting Lessons in Wound Healing." *Bulletin of the History of Medicine* 41 (March–April 1967): 97–131.

Wangensteen, Owen H.; Wangensteen, Sarah D.; and Klinger, Charles F. "Some Pre-Listerian and Post-Listerian Antiseptic Wound Practices and the Emergence of Asepsis." *Surgery, Gynecology & Obstetrics* 137 (October 1973): 677–702.

Wangensteen, Owen H., and Wangensteen, Sarah D. "Lister, His Books, and Evolvement of His Antiseptic Wound Practices." *Bulletin of the History of Medicine* 48 (Spring 1974): 100–28.

Warner, John Harley. "Therapeutic Explanation and the Edinburgh Bloodletting Controversy: Two Perspectives on the Medical Meaning of Science in the Mid-Nineteenth Century." *Medical History* 24 (July 1980): 241–58.

Young, Archibald. "Lord Lister's Life and Work." *Janus* 31 (May 1927): 318–35.

BOOKS

Ackerknecht, Erwin. *A Short History of Medicine.* rev. ed. Baltimore: The Johns Hopkins University Press, 1982.

Best, Edward. "Joseph Lister (1827–1912)." In *Mid-Nineteenth-Century Scientists,* pp. 139–72. Edited by John North. Oxford: Pergamon Press, 1969.

Bishop, W. J. *The Early History of Surgery.* New York: Barnes & Noble, Inc., 1960.

Brand, Jeanne L. *Doctors and the State: The British Medical Profession and Government Action in Public Health, 1870–1912.* Baltimore: The Johns Hopkins Press, 1965.

Brock, Thomas D. *Robert Koch: A Life in Medicine and Bacteriology.* Madison, Wisconsin: Science Tech Publishers, 1988.

Cameron, Hector Charles. *Joseph Lister: The Friend of Man.* London: William Heinemann, 1949.

Carter, K. Codell, trans. *Essays of Robert Koch.* New York: Greenwood Press, 1987.

Carter, K. Codell and Carter, Barbara R. *Childbed Fever: A Scientific Biography of Ignaz Semmel-weis.* Westport, Connecticut: Greenwood Press, 1994.

Cartwright, Frederick F. *Joseph Lister: The Man Who Made Surgery Safe.* London: Weidenfeld & Nicolson, 1963.

———. *The Development of Modern Surgery.* London: Arthur Barker Limited, 1967.

———. "Antiseptic Surgery." In *Medicine and Science in the 1860s,* pp. 77–103. Edited by F. N. L. Poynter. London: Wellcome Institute for the History of Medicine, 1968.

Checkland, Olive. "Local government and the health environment." In *Health Care as Social History: The Glasgow Case,* p. 12. Edited by Olive Checkland and Margaret Lamb. Aberdeen, Scotland: Aberdeen University Press, 1982.

Cheyne, W. Watson. *Lister and His Achievement.* London: Longmans, Green and Co., 1925.

Coleman, James S.; Katz, Elihu; and Menzel, Herbert. *Medical Innovation: A Diffusion Study.* Indianapolis: The Bobbs-Merrill Company, Inc., 1966.

Crellin, J. K. "The Dawn of the Germ Theory: Particles, Infection and Biology." In *Medicine and Science in the 1860s,* pp. 57–76. Edited by F. N. L. Poynter. London: Wellcome Institute for the History of Medicine, 1968.

Crowther, M. A. *The Workhouse System, 1834–1929: The History of an English Social Institution.* Athens, Georgia: The University of Georgia Press, 1981.

Dolan, John P., and Adams-Smith, William N. *Health and Society: A Documentary History of Medicine.* New York: The Seabury Press, 1978.

Dubos, Rene. *Pasteur and Modern Science.* London: Heinemann, 1960.

Dukes, Cuthbert. *Lord Lister (1827–1912).* London: Leonard Parsons, 1924.

Eyler, John M. *Victorian Social Medicine: The Ideas and Methods of William Farr.* Baltimore: The Johns Hopkins University Press, 1979.

Fisher, Richard B. *Joseph Lister, 1827–1912.* New York: Stein and Day, 1977.

French, Richard D. *Antivivisection and Medical Science in Victorian Society.* Princeton, New Jersey: Princeton University Press, 1975.

Gaskell, E. "Medical Literature." In *Medicine and Science in the 1860s,* pp. 289–309. Edited by F. N. L. Poynter. London: Wellcome Institute for the History of Medicine, 1968.

Godlee, Rickman John. *Lord Lister.* 3d ed. Oxford: The Clarendon Press, 1924.

Gordon, Richard. *Great Medical Disasters.* New York: Stein and Day, 1983; reprint ed., New York: Dorset Press, 1986.

Granshaw, Lindsay. "'Upon this Principle I have based a Practice': The Development and Reception of Antisepsis in Britain, 1867–90." In *Medical Innovations in Historical Perspective,* pp. 17–46. Edited by John V. Pickstone. New York: St. Martin's Press, 1992.

Guthrie, Douglas. *From Witchcraft to Antisepsis: A Study in Antithesis.* Lawrence, Kansas: University of Kansas Press, 1955.

Haeger, Knut. *The Illustrated History of Surgery.* New York: Bell Publishing Company, 1988.

Haggard, Howard W. *The Doctor in History.* New York: Dorset Press, 1989.

Haley, Bruce. *The Healthy Body and Victorian Culture.* Cambridge, Massachusetts: Harvard University Press, 1978.

Hamilton, David, and Lamb, Margaret. "Surgeons and surgery." In *Health Care as Social History: The Glasgow Case,* pp. 74–85. Edited by Olive Checkland and Margaret Lamb. Aberdeen, Scotland: Aberdeen University Press, 1982.

Hibbert, Christopher, ed. *Queen Victoria in her Letters and Journals.* New York: Viking, 1984.

Hodgkinson, Ruth G. "Social Medicine and the Growth of Statistical Information." In *Medicine and Science in the 1860s,* pp. 183–98. Edited by F. N. L. Poynter. London: Wellcome Institute for the History of Medicine, 1968.

Kargon, Robert H. *Science in Victorian Manchester.* Baltimore: The Johns Hopkins University Press, 1977.

Krause, Richard M. *The Restless Tide: The Persistent Challenge of the Microbial World.* Washington, D.C.: The National Foundation for Infectious Diseases, 1981.

Kuhn, Thomas S. *The Structure of Scientific Revolutions.* Chicago: The University of Chicago Press, 1962.

Lambert, Samuel W., and Goodwin, George M. *Medical Leaders from Hippocrates to Osler.* Indianapolis: The Bobbs-Merrill Company, 1929.

Lawrence, Christopher, and Dixey, Richard. "Practising on Principle: Joseph Lister and the Germ Theories of Disease." In *Medical Theory, Surgical Practice,* pp. 153–215. Edited by Christopher Lawrence. London: Routledge, 1992.

MacLeod, Roy M. "The Anatomy of State Medicine: Concept and Application." In *Medicine and Science in the 1860s,* pp. 199–227. Edited by F. N. L. Poynter. London: Wellcome Institute for the History of Medicine, 1968.

MacNalty, Arthur Salusbury. *A Biography of Sir Benjamin Ward Richardson.* London: Harvey & Blythe, Ltd., 1950.

Magner, Lois. *A History of Medicine.* New York: Marcel Dekker, Inc., 1992.

Miles, Alexander. *The Edinburgh School of Surgery before Lister.* London: A. & C. Black, Ltd., 1918.

———. "Before the Dawn." In *Joseph, Baron Lister: Centenary Volume, 1827–1927,* pp. 25–39. Edited by A. Logan Turner. Edinburgh: Oliver and Boyd, 1927.

Morris, James A. "The Royal Infirmary Buildings." In *Lister & the Lister Ward,* pp. 40–55. Glasgow: Jackson, Wylie and Co., 1927.

Morris, R. J. *Cholera, 1832: The Social Response to an Epidemic.* New York: Holmes & Meier Publishers, 1976.

Nuland, Sherwin B. *Doctors: The Biography of Medicine.* New York: Alfred A. Knopf, 1988.

Owen, David. *The Government of Victorian London, 1855–1889: The Metropolitan Board of Works, the Vestries, and the City Corporation.* Cambridge, Massachusetts: The Belknap Press of Harvard University Press, 1982.

Paget, Stephen. *Pasteur and After Pasteur.* London: Adam and Charles Black, 1914.

Pelling, Margaret. *Cholera, Fever and English Medicine, 1825–1865.* Oxford: Oxford University Press, 1978.

Peterson, M. Jeanne. *The Medical Profession in Mid-Victorian London.* Berkeley: University of California Press, 1978.

Rogers, Everett M. *Diffusion of Innovations.* New York: The Free Press, 1962.

Rosenberg, Charles E. *Explaining Epidemics and Other Studies in the History of Medicine.* Cambridge: Cambridge University Press, 1992.

Rupke, Nicolaas A. "Pro-vivisection in England in the Early 1880s: Arguments and Motives." In *Vivisection in Historical Perspective,* pp. 188–208. Edited by Nicolaas A. Rupke. London: Croom Helm, 1987.

Shepherd, John. "Lister and the Development of Abdominal Surgery." In *Medicine and Science in the 1860s,* pp. 105–115. Edited by F. N. L. Poynter. London: Wellcome Institute for the History of Medicine, 1968.

———. *Lawson Tait: The Rebellious Surgeon (1845–1899).* Lawrence, Kansas: Coronado Press, 1980.

Smith, F. B. *The People's Health, 1830–1910.* New York: Holmes & Meier Publishers, Inc., 1979.

The Research Readers of the Scientific Department, comp. *Lister and the Ligature.* New Brunswick, N.J.: Johnson & Johnson, 1925.

Towers, Bernard. "The Impact of Darwin's *Origin of Species* on Medicine and Biology." In *Medicine and Science in the 1860s,* pp. 45–55. Edited by F. N. L. Poynter. London: Wellcome Institute for the History of Medicine, 1968.

Vallery-Radot, Rene. *The Life of Pasteur.* Garden City, New York: Doubleday, Page & Company, 1926.

Vandervliet, Glenn. *Microbiology and the Spontaneous Generation Debate During the 1870's.* Lawrence, Kansas: Coronado Press, 1971.

Waddington, Ivan. "General Practitioners and Consultants in Early Nineteenth-Century England: The Sociology of an Intra-Professional Conflict." In *Health Care and Popular Medicine in Nineteenth Century England,* pp. 164–88. Edited by John Woodward and David Richards. New York: Holmes & Meier Publishers, 1977.

————. *The Medical Profession in the Industrial Revolution.* Dublin: Gill and Macmillan Humanities Press, 1984.

Williams, Guy. *The Age of Miracles: Medicine and Surgery in the Nineteenth Century.* London: Constable, 1981.

Wohl, Anthony S. *Endangered Lives: Public Health in Victorian Britain.* Cambridge, Massachusetts: Harvard University Press, 1983.

Woodward, John. *To do the sick no harm: A study of the British voluntary hospital system to 1875.* London: Routledge & Kegan Paul, 1974.

Wrench, G. T. *Lord Lister: His Life and Work.* New York: Frederick A. Stokes Company, 1914.

Youngson, A. J. *The Scientific Revolution in Victorian Medicine.* New York: Holmes & Meier Publishers, Inc., 1979.

MANUSCRIPTS

Kunz, Hubert. "The Reasons for Theodor Billroth's Initially Negative Attitude against Joseph Lister's Antiseptic Method." TMs. Lister Papers, Royal College of Surgeons of England, London, Drawer 2, Envelope 2.

Index

free trade, 17, 22–23
fungi, 21, 36, 64–65, 68, 70, 75

Gairdner, William, 18
Gamgee, Sampson, 34, 92–93
Gladstone, William, 133
Glover, James Grey, 118
Godlee, Rickman J., 60, 106, 119
Goodyear Rubber Company, 124
Gould, A. Pearce, 118
governmental agencies
    Army Medical Department, 12
    Army Sanitary Commission, 12
    General Board of Health, 20, 23, 26
    General Council of Medical Education and
        Registration, 8
    General Register Office, 13
    Indian Sanitary Commission, 12
    Local Governmnent Board, 27
    Medical Officers of Health, 20, 27
    Poor Law Administration, 27
    Poor Law Commission, 20
    Privy Council, 26, 76
Granshaw, Lindsay, 55
Grant, President, 108
Great Stink, 26
Greenlees, James, 30
Gross, Samuel, 108–109

Hair, Philip, 34
Halsted, William Stewart, 124
Harley, George, 88–89
Hart, Ernest, 127, 131, 133
Harvey, William, 15
Haydon, William, 59
Heath, Christopher, 103
Hensman, Arthur, 35–36
Holmes, Timothy, 102–103, 113–115, 120,
    128–130
hospitals
    Belfast General, 41
    Belgrave Hospital for Children, 102
    Birmingham General, 54
    Charing-Cross, 40, 103
    Charite, 100, 124
    county, 13
    Glasgow Fever, 88
    Guy's, 8, 38–39, 62, 95, 104, 111–112, 115
    Johns Hopkins University, 124
    King's College, 33, 39, 61, 109–111, 113, 123
    large, 2, 11, 31, 43, 60, 112
    London, 37, 54
    lying-in, 10
    metropolitan, 1, 13, 62–63, 103, 112
    Middlesex, 37, 54

military, 12
    National Hospital of the Epileptic and Para-
        lysed, 66
    North-Eastern Hospital for Children, 58
    provincial, 13, 119
    Richmond, 118
    Royal Hospital for Diseases of the Chest, 58
    salubrity of, 49, 51
    Samaritan Free Hospital for Women and Chil-
        dren, 125
    small, 1, 38, 60
    St. Bartholomew's, 38–39, 62, 103, 106, 116,
        119–120
    St. George's, 37, 54, 103
    St. John's Hospital for Skin Diseases, 69
    St. Mary's, 54–55
    St. Thomas's, 12, 119, 121
    The Queen's Hospital, 92, 121
    University College, 40, 60, 66, 103–104, 116
    University of Aberdeen, 34
    University of Edinburgh, 40
    Victoria Hospital for Children, 59
    Vienna General, 10
Howse, H. G., 112, 115
Hunter, John, 3
Huxley, Thomas, 66
hygiene, 60, 69
    cleanliness, 17, 116–117, 121, 123–125, 128,
        134
    sanitation, 12, 14, 20, 24, 39, 43, 69

implements
    chain saw, 4
    cutting pliers, 123–124
    drainage tubes, 42, 55, 92, 97–98, 100, 117,
        122, 125–126, 134
    dressing scissors, 98
    forceps, 6, 30, 61, 97
    mackintosh, 55, 96, 125
    sponges, 10, 12, 47, 98, 125
    wicks, 42
Indian Mutiny, 12
India rubber, 42, 55, 97, 100, 122, 126
industrialization, 8–9, 41
infirmaries
    Aberdeen Royal, 129
    Edinburgh Royal, 3, 9, 43–44, 96, 100–101
    Glasgow Royal, 8–9, 14, 47–52, 95, 105, 117,
        124
    Kidderminster, 40
    Leeds General, 44
    Liverpool Royal, 43
    Poor Law, 28
    voluntary, 9